Pediatric Transillumination

Pediatric Transillumination

Steven M. Donn, M.D.
Assistant Professor
Department of Pediatrics
Section of Newborn Services
University of Michigan Medical School
Ann Arbor, Michigan

Lawrence R. Kuhns, M.D.
Clinical Professor
Department of Radiology
University of Michigan Medical School
Ann Arbor, Michigan

YEAR BOOK MEDICAL PUBLISHERS, INC.
CHICAGO • LONDON

Library of Congress Cataloging in Publication Data

Donn, Steven M.
  Pediatric transillumination.

  Bibliography: p.
  Includes index.
  1. Infants (Newborn)—Diseases—Diagnosis.
2. Transillumination. I. Kuhns, Lawrence R. II. Title.
[DNLM: 1. Transillumination—In infancy and childhood.
WS 141 D685p]
RJ255.6.T7D66   1982   618.92'01   82-11035
ISBN 0-8151-2733-2

Contributors

RAUL C. BANAGALE, M.D.
Assistant Professor, Department of Pediatrics, Section of Newborn Services, University of Michigan Medical School; Director of Nurseries, St. Joseph Mercy Hospital, Ann Arbor, Michigan

STEVEN M. DONN., M.D.
Assistant Professor, Department of Pediatrics, Section of Newborn Services, University of Michigan Medical School, Ann Arbor, Michigan

BRIAN J. DUCHINSKY, M.S.
Computed Tomography Field Service Development Engineer, General Electric Medical Systems, Milwaukee, Wisconsin

LAWRENCE R. KUHNS, M.D.
Clinical Professor, Department of Radiology, University of Michigan Medical School, Ann Arbor, Michigan

JOAQUIN O. UY, M.D., Ph.D.
Department of Radiology/Nuclear Medicine, Mercy Hospital, Monroe, Michigan

To Paula, Elaine, and Richard
and
To Jane, Matt, Liz, Brian, and Tim

Contents

PART II   CLINICAL TRANSILLUMINATION
S. M. Donn, M.D., and L. R. Kuhns, M.D.

COLOR PLATES

PART III   APPENDICES

Foreword

ANYONE WHO HAS experienced the quantum leap in the power of imaging brought about by computerized tomography and ultrasonography in recent years might agree to call this the age of noninvasive diagnostics. Indeed, even more powerful (and technically more demanding) methods, such as positron emission tomography and nuclear magnetic resonance, will make us leap again. Against this background of "modern" advances stands the renewed interest in the diagnostic use of transillumination with visible light. The present volume summarizes what has been learned about the clinical use of transillumination, predominantly in newborn infants.

This book will have been most useful if it stimulates refinement and further application of transillumination as a means of rapid, noninvasive, inexpensive bedside evaluation and clinical enlightenment.

DIETRICH W. ROLOFF, M.D.
Associate Professor of Pediatrics
Director of Newborn Services
The University of Michigan Hospitals

Preface

TRANSILLUMINATION has been applied to clinical medicine for over 150 years. However, the more recent growth in the techniques of transillumination has paralleled that of neonatology owing to its many uses in the newborn. Its use in clinical practice has become widespread in nurseries because of its reliability, noninvasiveness, and minimal expense. It has been applied to several organs and anatomical regions and is considered by many to have become a first-line diagnostic tool.

It is the purpose of this volume to acquaint the reader with the scientific principles of transillumination and its use in the practice of pediatrics. We have divided the book into three sections.

Part I deals with the basics of transillumination. Chapter 1 describes the history of transillumination in medicine, reviewing the major developments since Richard Bright's first description. Chapter 2 presents the principles of transillumination, including the nature of light, its interaction with matter, and its filtration. Chapter 3 summarizes equipment and principles of measurement, including available light sources and light meters.

Part II is devoted to clinical transillumination. Chapter 4 describes the general techniques of pediatric transillumination. This is followed by a regional atlas which reviews normal and abnormal findings in the transillumination of the head and neck (chapter 5), chest (chapter 6), abdomen and spine (chapter 7), and extremities and blood vessels (chapter 8). We have included a section of color reproductions to illustrate some of the more striking diagnoses which we have encountered using transillumination under optimal lighting conditions.

Part III contains a further description of some physical aspects of light and its measurement, and defines related terminology. Additionally, there is an extensive bibliography of transillumination which includes both pediatric and adult applications.

It is hoped that the reader will not only become familiar with the many applications of transillumination, but also may realize the tremendous potential for the use of light in medicine.

ACKNOWLEDGMENTS

The preparation of this book would not have been possible without the contributions of the staffs of the Holden Neonatal Intensive Care Unit and C. S. Mott Children's Hospital, The University of Michigan Hospitals. We would like to thank the many nurses, respiratory therapists, radiology technologists, house officers, fellows, and staff physicians whose efforts were paramount in the development of many of the applications of transillumination.

We would like to acknowledge the efforts of Dr. John Cameron, Medical Physics Division, University of Wisconsin, for his collaboration on many transillumination projects and his efforts in promoting the design and production of several pieces of equipment which have furthered transillumination.

Special thanks are in order for Mrs. Betty Passon, who prepared the entire manuscript, and Dr. Raul C. Banagale for his excellent photographic contributions, and for Kenneth E. Hoppens of Year Book Medical Publishers for his support and encouragement of this project.

STEVEN M. DONN, M.D.
LAWRENCE R. KUHNS, M.D.

Part I

BASICS OF
TRANSILLUMINATION

1

History of Transillumination

R. C. Banagale, M.D.

Be not the first to lay the old aside, nor yet the last by whom the new are try'd.
—Alexander Pope

TRANSILLUMINATION, the passage of light rays through the tissues and cavities of the body, was first introduced as a viable diagnostic aid in the early nineteenth century. Crude utilization of various sources of light, including that of candles and, in some instances, direct sunlight, enabled the examiner to determine gross abnormalities in shape, substance, and relative density of an organ, tumor, or other object of his study.

Over the course of the next one hundred fifty years tremendous advances were made in the techniques of transillumination. Candlelight was supplanted by fiberoptic transilluminators, and the techniques used to detect gross irregularities were categorically refined to provide not only specific diagnostic comprehension, but also versatile therapeutic assistance.

APPLICATION AND CLINICAL EXPERIENCE

Transillumination of the Head

Transillumination of the head (Fig 1-1) was first described in 1831 by Richard Bright:

James Cardinal, aged 29, was admitted into Guy's Hospital under the care of Sir Astley Cooper, December 1st, 1824. . . . [H]is head was at least twice the size which his spare body would lead us to expect. . . . If a candle was held behind his head, or the sun happened to be behind it, the cranium appeared semi-transparent.

It was not until 1910, however, that what Bright recorded as an observation would first be used to pursue specific medical information. In that year Strasburger recorded the performance of cranial transillumination on a 3-month-old hydrocephalic infant, using a lamp positioned behind the baby's head. Von Bokay, in 1913, reported his utilization of basically the same technique on 15 children with a diagnosis of chronic hydrocephalus internus. He published his further experiences in a systematic use of transillumination in 1915, 1923, and 1932.

The introduction of ventriculography in 1921 by Dandy as a more precise procedure in locating the exact site and character of an obstruction in a hydrocephalic patient briefly encroached on the burgeoning popularity of transillumination as a beneficial tool. However, in 1950 Hamby and his associates presented seven cases of hydranencephaly and reemphasized the value of cranial transillumination as the single simplest and most valuable aid in diagnosis. They described their experience relative to one of the hydranencephalic children:

The head was held in the beam of a strong light in a darkened room. A remarkable picture was seen. . . . The entire cranium glowed with an orange-red light like an illuminated Japanese lantern. When the beam was directed against the occiput and the eyelids were held open, the glow was transmitted clearly through the pupils. . . . Opacities could be seen representing the major cranial buttresses, the large scalp veins and the superior longitudinal sinus.

Alexander and associates (1956), feeling that the value of cranial transillumination was being somewhat neglected by neurologists and pediatricians, published an article which described a contrivance by which more precise transillumination would be possible. They devised a table apparatus upon which an infant could be placed with his head over an opening, illuminated from below by a 100-watt bulb. A 2-inch-thick foam rubber pad around the opening was shaped so as to fit the patient's head and, at the same time, prevent the escape of light around it. As an added feature, the apparatus was capable of taking both black and white and color photographs of the transilluminated head. This device is described in better detail by Taylor and his co-workers in a later report (Taylor et al., 1956).

In 1958 Horner and colleagues presented a very simple modification of cranial transillumination during the Sixty-Eighth Annual Meeting of the American Pediatric Society, which Horner restated in a later publication (1962). He described the use of a standard two-cell flashlight with a narrow cuff of opaque sponge rubber surrounding the illuminating surface. In a darkened room the cuff is pressed against the cra-

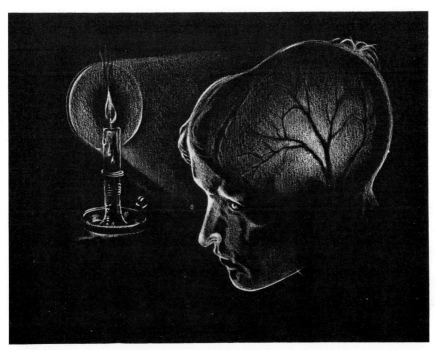

Fig 1–1.—Artist's interpretation of Richard Bright's observation of the transillumination of the head of James Cardinal, 1831. (Drawing by Lewis Sadler.)

nial vault allowing the foam rubber to conform to the contours of the skull surface. The extent of the rim of light around the rubber cone is observed.

Dodge, who participated in the discussion of Horner's 1958 presentation, also published with Porter his experience utilizing basically the same technique (1961). In addition, numerous other works demonstrating the value of cranial transillumination in cranial and intracranial pathology were published (Calliauw, 1962; Shurtleff, 1964; Lehman et al., 1970; Rozovski et al., 1971; Nixon et al., 1974; and Haller, 1981). These dealt with hydrocephalus of varied etiology, subdural hygroma, hydranencephaly, subdural effusion, cystic disease of the brain, porencephaly, scalp edema, subdural hematoma, and the observation of increased transillumination in severely malnourished infants.

The detracting aspect common to all methods of transillumination up to this point was the need for a completely dark room. Lack of provision for this within the hospital unit, coupled with the difficulty of holding a squirming infant or moving an acutely ill newborn, necessitated technological refinements.

One form these refinements took was that of a Pulsed Transilluminator* for cranial transillumination, which was first introduced by Hayden et al. in 1975. The pulsed transilluminator contains a gallium arsenide infrared emitting diode and a silicon photodetector diode. The light emitter and detector are built into one hand-held unit which can be firmly placed on the infant's head. A meter is calibrated to read the transmitted infrared intensity in optical density units per centimeter (OD/cm).

In the same year, Cheldelin and his colleagues (1975) reported the use of the Chun Gun,† named in honor of Dr. Ray Chun of the University of Wisconsin Medical School, who was instrumental in its development. Using the Chun Gun with a standardized light source and absorbing filters, they reported normal values for cranial transillumination.

In 1976, Swick et al. reported transillumination values for premature infants, also with the use of the Chun Gun. The procedure was done in a totally darkened room and calipers were used to measure the extent of transillumination. They found, with increasing gestational age, a progressive increase in transillumination over three sites: the anterior fontanelle, the frontotemporal fossa, and the parieto-occipital eminence.

In 1977, Vyhmeister and associates reported their experience with the use of a Chun Gun that had been fitted with a flexible plastic disk‡ to simplify the measurement of transillumination. They pointed out the impracticality of completely darkening the room and performed the procedure in controlled, subdued light. An important difference between their findings and those of Swick is the observation of a progressive increase in transillumination with increasing gestational age only in the occipital region.

The use of high-intensity transillumination in detecting a growing skull fracture in an 8-month-old female infant was reported by Kuhns et al. (1977). Further experience with the use of a fiberoptic device‖ and a cadmium sulfide light meter§ in detecting neonatal intracranial hemorrhage was reported by Donn and associates (1979).

During the course of the development of transilluminating instru-

---

*Center for BioEngineering, University of Washington, Seattle, WA.
†Radiation Measurements, Inc., Middleton, WI.
‡Audio-Visual Department, Loma Linda, CA.
‖Omni-Source Med General, Inc., Minneapolis, MN.
§TLM 2, Radiation Measurements, Inc., Middleton, WI.

ments and techniques, many attempts have been made to record permanently the findings on transillumination devices. The apparatus for photography and transillumination of the head devised by Taylor and his colleagues (1956) is no longer practical with the present-day set-up in the neonatal intensive care unit. In 1961, Cambern and associates described their technique of cranial transillumination photography; however, their experience was before the availability of high-speed color film. In 1966, Shurtleff and associates described transillumination photography using a 200-watt second strobe, triggered by a photocell, as fill light with a blue filter bounced from ceiling or wall.

Martin and co-workers (1977) described a technique of transillumination photography in the radiographic rooms using 35-mm film that can be processed in an automatic x-ray processor.

Transillumination of the Chest

A very early attempt to apply transillumination to the tissues of the chest was made by the Scottish physician, Sir James Simpson, in 1869. Fostered by the development of the electric incandescent light, Simpson examined the famous Siamese twins, Eng and Chang, conjoined by a band of tissue from sternum to sternum. Simpson wrote:

You are well aware that various attempts have been made of late years, by electric and other strong lights, to make portions of the body more or less translucent. By placing a powerful light behind the connecting band in Eng and Chang, I tried to make its thinner portions transparent, with a view of possibly tracing its contents better than by touch; but I failed entirely in getting any advantage from this mode of examination.

One of the first applications of transillumination as a diagnostic tool in diseases involving the chest was reported by Cutler in 1929 when he reported on the value of transillumination in the diagnosis and interpretation of pathologic conditions in the breast:

Transillumination is of special value in those cases of bleeding nipple in which no tumor can be palpated. In these cases, in which localization of the lesion has heretofore been difficult or impossible, transillumination usually enables localization of the lesion and thereby directly indicates the site for operative removal.

The value of transillumination in the diagnosis of chest abnormalities in infants did not receive wide attention until 1975 when experience was reported by Kuhns and colleagues. A high-intensity transilluminator, the Mini-Light Portable Illuminator,* was utilized successfully in

---

*Med General, Minneapolis, MN.

diagnosing neonatal pneumothorax or pneumomediastinum. The tip of the flexible 5-foot fiberoptic light probe was adapted for transillumination by placing a piece of soft black rubber tubing over it.

In 1977, pediatric surgeons (Buck et al., 1977) reported their own clinical experience utilizing fiberoptic transillumination not only for thoracic pathology but also for the applications of transillumination to other anatomical locations. This procedure has been particularly advantageous in cases of diaphragmatic hernia where pneumothorax is a common complication.

Heat buildup in the skin during high-intensity transillumination did, at one time, limit the duration of its application. However, Uy and associates (1977) corrected this problem with the use of a glass filter blank,* which filters light with wavelengths below 570 nm, placed in front of the quartz-iodide lamp of the illuminator. Scanlon (1977) recommended the use of a swan-bill-shaped black lamb's nipple† with the feeding hole end cut to slide over the fiberoptic tip to help reduce heat buildup. Very recently, Bellotti and co-workers (1981) constructed a simple shield to absorb heat at the tip of the fiberoptic cable utilizing a modified blood pressure monitor transducer dome. The shield is filled with either clear or red-dyed polyester casting resin. An opening in the center of the resin permits fitting the shield onto the end of the light cable.

Transillumination of the Abdomen and Pelvis

In 1843, a few years after Bright's account of skull transillumination, Curling described the transillumination of a hydrocele utilizing a lighted candle and with the tumor interposed between the surgeon and the light:

When examined by transmitted light, the tumor is found to be more or less transparent, except at the part where the testis is situated, the opacity there indicating the exact position of the gland.

He also described the earliest modification in enhancing the clinical observation during transillumination:

I have sometimes derived considerable assistance from using a wooden tube, about three quarters of an inch in diameter, open at both extremities. One end being placed against the swelling opposite the light, the surgeon, on looking

---

*CS-2-73 Corning, F.J. Gray Co., Jamaica, NY.
†No. 97, Davol Inc., Providence, RI.

through the other, can observe the transparency with great advantage. If a more convenient tube be not at hand, a roll of writing paper will answer the same purpose.

Altchek described the value of transillumination in gynecologic examinations with special application in the diagnosis of vesicovaginal fistula (1962) and enterocele (1965).

In 1966, Kravitz et al. described the use of bright light shone through umbilical cords as a methodological adjunct in screening and early detection of cases of single umbilical artery in the newborn. Wide application of abdominal transillumination in the newborn, however, did not receive great acceptance until 1966, when Shurtleff and associates described the utilization of the procedure on a 4-month-old infant with marked ascites who eventually was found to have a congenital stenosis of the mesenteric vein.

In 1968, Mofenson and Greensher emphasized the usefulness of transillumination in detecting abdominal masses in infants. Their brief report consisted of several cases, which included urinary bladder distention, multicystic kidneys, hydronephrosis, retroperitoneal teratoma, perirenal cyst, ascites, and bowel distention secondary to intestinal atresia.

Wedge and co-workers (1971) reported a ten-year clinical experience with 63 cases of abdominal masses in children wherein the value of abdominal transillumination, as part of routine physical examination, was emphasized.

In the mid 1970s, reports (Wyman and Kuhns, 1976; Buck et al., 1977) were published demonstrating the utilization of fiberoptic transillumination in the diagnosis of pneumoperitoneum, ascites, hydronephrosis, sacrococcygeal teratoma, and intra-abdominal cysts. It was also found to facilitate suprapubic aspiration of the urine and the placement of oroduodenal tubes in the newborn.

Transillumination of the Extremities

The technique of transillumination as an untapped resource to aid in starting intravenous infusions has been available since the inception of intravenous therapy. Latta described the early use of venipuncture and intravenous injection of saline into adult patients suffering from cholera in 1831, the same year Bright first described the principle of transillumination. Karelitz (1931, 1934) described the extensive use of intravenous infusion in children about one hundred years later.

It was not until the mid-1970s, however, that transillumination was used as a valuable adjunct in intravenous line insertion. Gerbitz (1974) reported the usefulness of the fiberoptic transilluminator as a handy tool for nurses locating veins for venipuncture. Physicans and nurses involved in the care of ill newborns are aware of the difficulty in obtaining repeated blood samples by percutaneous venous or arterial puncture. This technical difficulty has been overcome, for the most part, by the use of transillumination.

Clinical experience with this technique was reported by Kuhns and associates (1975) and by Wall and Kuhns (1977). Cole et al. (1978) reported their own success in percutaneous cannulation of the radial artery in the newborn with the use of a fiberoptic transilluminator.

The usefulness of transillumination was also reported by Goldman and colleagues (1977) in the diagnosis of digital mucinous pseudocysts.

Other Applications of Transillumination

In 1867, Bruck described his experience with the use of a stomatoscope in the transillumination of the teeth and neighboring regions.

Cameron, in the 1922 edition of his monograph entitled "Diagnosis by Transillumination," described the results of years of study on the use of transillumination in the diagnosis of infected conditions of the dental process and various air sinuses. He was instrumental in the development of an efficient 100-candlepower transilluminator called the Dentalamp, which was based on the searchlight principle. He wrote:

Searchlights are being constructed for commercial purposes which visibly project light a distance of five to eight miles by means of a powerful lamp, reflector and lens which concentrate the rays so that the light is projected in one beam parallel to the axis . . . and after a great deal of laboratory work, this principle was applied in the development of a diagnostic lamp that makes diagnosis by transillumination a reality.

Further advances in technology and the common use of fiberoptics (Bomba, 1971; Taylor et al., 1967; Evans et al., 1975) enhanced the role of transillumination as a diagnostic tool relative to the oral cavity and air sinuses.

Cohen and colleagues (1975) reported the value of transillumination in locating the angular and frontal veins for orbital venography, thus enabling the surgeon to establish the locations of these veins to avoid cutting them during lacrimal sac procedures.

Goldman (1976) found transillumination a very helpful prebiopsy procedure for suspected basal carcinoma. He claimed that the optical characteristics of skin are changed by cords of basal cells infiltrating the dermis. The cords make for better transmission of light, especially when applied through the lip, cheek, and ear areas, and through the nose. He hopes that the reliability and efficiency of the technique can be perfected through the use of laser, helium-neon, and infrared technology.

Transillumination has also been used in ophthalmology. Peyman and Sanders (1975) have developed a scleral-indentor illuminator for better visualization of choroidal lesions. Cohen and associates (1976) have described transillumination biomicroscopical examination of the anterior chamber angle of the iris. It provided for high-intensity retroillumination to the anterior and posterior segments of the globe without producing heat. Experiences with dacryo-transillumination (Cohen, 1967), transillumination photography of the eye (Lichter, 1972), and infrared transillumination stereophotography (Saari et al., 1977) have been reported.

The techniques of intracardiac transillumination for detecting cardiac anomalies have also been published (Bernhard et al., 1962; Rosenquist et al., 1970; Daneshwar et al., 1979).

CONCLUSION

The principle of transillumination was first described in 1831. But, because of the procedure's inherent dependency on the general technological advancements of the time, it has taken more than 150 years to evolve into the valuable diagnostic and therapeutic aid of today. The fiberoptic transilluminators and highly specialized photographic equipment which have become integral parts of the modern medical regimen are a far cry from the use of candles, direct sunlight, and "camera mounted onto apparatus." However, while some of the crude initial instruments and methods described within this brief history may seem hopelessly archaic, it should not be forgotten that they were the forerunners of the highly refined system so widely in use today.

REFERENCES

Alexander E., et al.: Hydranencephaly: Observations on transillumination of the head of infants. *Arch. Neurol. Psychiatr.* 76:578–584, 1956.

Altchek A.: Diagnosis of enterocele by negative intrarectal transillumination. *Obstet. Gynecol.* 26:636–639, 1965.

Altchek A.: Transillumination—a new method of vesicovaginal fistula investigation. *Obstet. Gynecol.* 20:458–461, 1962.

Bellotti G.A., et al.: Fiberoptic transillumination for intravenous cannulation under general anesthesia. *Anesth. Analg.* 60:348–351, 1981.

Bernhard W.F., et al.: Transillumination of the ventricular septum. *N. Engl. J. Med.* 267:909–912, 1962.

Bokay J.: Die strasburgersche transparenzuntersuchung bei chronischem hydrocephalus internus. *Jahrb. Kinderheilkd.* 78:426–441, 1913.

Bokay J.: Beitrage zur pathologie und therapie des chronischen hydrocephalus internus. *Jahrb. Kinderheilkd.* 81:17–24, 1915.

Bokay J.: Neue beitrage zun wert der transparenzuntersuchung nach strasburger bei chronischem hydrocephalus internus. *Monatsschr. Kinderheilkd.* 24:43, 1923.

Bokay J.: Über den Wert der transparenzuntersuchungen bei hydrocephalus internus congenitus. *Acta Paediatr.* 13:48, 1932.

Bomba J.L.: Fiberoptic lighting systems: Their role in dentistry. *Dent. Clin. North Am.* 15:197–218, 1971.

Bright R.: Diseases of the brain and nervous system, in *Reports of Medical Cases Selected With a View of Illustrating the Symptoms and Cure of Diseases by a Reference to Morbid Anatomy.* London, Logman, Rees, Orme, Brown and Green, and Highley, 1831, vol. 2, case CCV.

Bruck J.: *Das Urethroscop und das Stomatoscop zur Durchleuchtung der Blase und der Zähne und ihrer Nachbartheile durch galvanisches Glühlicht.* Breslau, Maruschke & Berendt, 1867.

Buck J.R., et al.: Fiberoptic transillumination—a new tool for the pediatric surgeon. *J. Pediatr. Surg.* 12:451–463, 1977.

Calliauw L.: The value of transillumination of the skull in neurological examination of neonates and infants. *Acta Neurochir.* 10:75–91, 1961.

Cambern A.M., et al.: Photography of transilluminated intracranial lesions in infants. *Med. Radiogr. Photogr.* 37:8–11, 1961.

Cameron W.J.: *Diagnosis by Transillumination,* ed 3. Chicago, Cameron's Publishing Co., 1922.

Cheldelin L.V., et al.: Normal values for transillumination of skull using a new light source. *J. Pediatr.* 87:937–938, 1975.

Cohen S.W.: Dacryo-transillumination. *Am. J. Ophthalmol.* 63:127–128, 1967.

Cohen S.W., et al.: Transillumination of the angular and frontal veins. *Am. J. Ophthalmol.* 80:765–766, 1975.

Cohen S.W., et al.: Biomicroscopical choroidoscopy (uveoscopy) and transillumination gonioscopy. *Arch. Ophthalmol.* 94:1618–1621, 1976.

Cole F.S., et al.: Technique for percutaneous cannulation of the radial artery in the newborn infant. *J. Pediatr.* 92:105–107, 1978.

Curling T.B.: Hydrocele, in Goddard P.B., (ed.): *A Practical Treatise on the Diseases of the Testis, and of the Spermatic Cord and Scrotum.* Philadelphia, Carey and Hart, 1843, chap. 4.

Cutler M: Transillumination as an aid in the diagnosis of breast lesions. *Surg. Gynecol. Obstet.* 48:721–729, 1929.

Dandy W.E.: The diagnosis and treatment of hydrocephalus due to occlusions of the foramina of Magendie and Luschka. *Surg. Gynecol. Obstet.* 23:112–124, 1921.

Daneshwar A., et al.: Transventricular illumination. *Ann. Thorac. Surg.* 28:94–95, 1979.

Dodge P.R., Porter P.: Demonstration of intracranial pathology by transillumination. *Arch. Neurol.* 5:30–41, 1961.

Donn S.M., et al.: Rapid detection of neonatal intracranial hemorrhage by transillumination. *Pediatrics* 64:843–847, 1979.

Evans F.O., et al.: Sinusitis of the maxillary antrum. *N. Engl. J. Med.* 293:735–739, 1975.

Gerbitz S.: Transillumination helps nurses locate veins. *Nursing* 4:12, 1974.

Goldman J.A., et al.: Digital mucinous pseudocysts. *Arthritis Rheum.* 20:997–1002, 1977.

Goldman L.: Transillumination as a diagnostic aid. *Arch. Dermatol.* 112:262, 1976.

Haller J.S.: Skull transillumination, in Coleman M.C. (ed.): *Neonatal Neurology.* Baltimore, University Park Press, 1981.

Hamby W.B., et al.: Hydranencephaly: Clinical diagnosis. *Pediatrics* 6:371–383, 1950.

Hayden P.W., et al.: A pulsed transilluminator for the infant cranium. *Clin. Pediatr.* 14:627–632, 1975.

Horner F.A.: The technique of transillumination of the skull. *Am. J. Dis. Child.* 103:183–184, 1962.

Horner F.A., et al.: Diagnosis of collection of subdural fluid by transillumination. *Am J. Dis. Child.* 96:594–595, 1958.

Karelitz S.: Continuous intravenous method of fluid administration (venoclysis) in pediatrics. *NY State J. Med.* 34:63–66, 1934.

Karelitz S., et al.: Treatment of toxicosis with the aid of a continuous intravenous drip of dextrose solution. *Am. J. Dis. Child.* 42:781–802, 1931.

Kravitz H., et al.: A technique for improved visualization of the umbilical vessels. *I.M.J.* 130:23–25, 1966.

Kuhns L.R., et al.: Intense transillumination for infant venipuncture. *Radiology* 116:734–735, 1975.

Kuhns L.R., et al.: Diagnosis of pneumothorax or pneumomediastinum in the neonate by transillumination. *Pediatrics* 56:355–360, 1975.

Kuhns L.R., et al.: Transillumination detection of a growing skull fracture. *Am J. Dis. Child* 131:889–892, 1977.

Latta T.: Treatment of cholera by the copius injection of aqueous and saline fluids into the veins. *Lancet* 18:274–277, 1831.

Lehman R.A.W., et al.: Cystic intracranial teratoma in an infant. *J. Neurosurg.* 33:334–338, 1970.

Lichter P.R.: Transillumination photography of the eye. *Am. J. Ophthalmol.* 73:927–931, 1972.

Martin A.J., et al.: Production of a permanent radiographic record of transillumination of the neonate. *Radiology* 122:540–541, 1977.

Mofenson H.C., Greensher J.: Transillumination of the abdomen in infants. *Am. J. Dis. Child.* 115:428–431, 1968.

Nixon G.W., et al.: Congenital porencephaly. *Pediatrics* 54:43–50, 1974.

Peyman G.A., Sanders D.R.: Transillumination ophthalmoscopy: Instrumentation and technique. *Ophthalmic. Surg.* 6:15–16, 1975.

Rosenquist G.C., et al.: Right atrial–left ventricular relationships in tricuspid atresia: Position of the presumed site of the atretic valve as determined by transillumination. *Am. Heart J.* 80:493–497, 1970.

Rozovski J.N., et al.: Cranial transillumination in early and severe malnutrition. *Br. J. Nutr.* 25:107–111, 1971.

Saari M., et al.: Infrared transillumination stereophotography of normal iris. *Can. J. Ophthal.* 12:308–311, 1977.

Scanlon J.W.: A modification of chest transilluminator. *Pediatrics* 60:766, 1977.

Shurtleff D.B.: Transillumination of skull in infants and children. *Am. J. Dis. Child.* 107:14–24, 1964.

Shurtleff D.B., et al.: Clinical use of transillumination. *Arch. Dis. Child.* 41:183–187, 1966.

Simpson J.: A lecture on the Siamese and other viable united twins. *Br. Med. J.*, i, 139, 1869.

Strasburger J.: Transparenz des kopies bei hydrocephalus. *Dtsch. Med. Wochenschr.* 36:294, 1910.

Swick H.M., et al.: Transillumination of the skull in premature infants. *Pediatrics* 58:658–664, 1976.

Taylor L., et al.: An apparatus for photography of transillumination of the head. *J. Neurosurg.* 13:219–220, 1956.

Taylor R.C., et al.: Illumination of the oral cavity. *J. Am. Dent. Assoc.* 74:1207–1209, 1967.

Uy J.O., et al.: Light filtration during transillumination of the neonate: A method to reduce heat buildup in the skin. *Pediatrics* 60:308–312, 1977.

Vyhmeister N., et al.: Cranial transillumination norms of the premature infant. *J. Pediatr.* 91:980–982, 1977.

Wall P.M., Kuhns L.R.: Percutaneous arterial sampling using transillumination. *Pediatrics* 59(suppl.):1032–1035, 1977.

Wedge J.J., et al.: Abdominal masses in the newborn: 63 cases. *J. Urol.* 106:770–775, 1971.

Wyman M.L., Kuhns L.R.: Pneumoperitoneum demonstrated by transillumination. *Am. J. Dis. Child.* 130:1237–1238, 1976.

2

Principles of Transillumination

J. O. Uy, M.D., Ph.D.

THE NATURE OF LIGHT

Light is described scientifically in two ways, as a wave and as a particle. The first is essential for a satisfactory explanation of phenomena such as interference and diffraction; the second is essential to the understanding of phenomena such as light absorption and photoelectric effect. Historically, the two descriptions have been considered in opposition and much intellectual energy has been expended in attempts to show that one was correct and the other wrong. The introduction of the electromagnetic theory by Maxwell in 1856 provided a strong quantitative foundation for the existence of radiation in the form of waves. In the early years of the twentieth century, it became evident that a particle description was necessary to explain certain phenomena and the concept of the photon arose. Much effort has been devoted to consideration of a "unified" description, in which particles and waves might be combined as different aspects of a single entity, but this approach has been unsuccessful.

Electromagnetic radiation ranges from gamma rays with wavelengths as short as 10^{-14} cm to radiowaves with wavelengths of thousands of meters. Visible light represents only a small portion of the electromagnetic radiation with wavelengths between 400 and 700 nanometers (Fig 2-1). Since light is a form of energy, its unit of measurement in wavelengths can be converted to energy units by using the following formula:

$$E = h\nu$$

15

where E is energy, h is Planck's constant, and v is wave frequency which is the inverse of wavelength. Applying the above formula, the electromagnetic radiation range can be converted to energy units such as electron volts (ev) (see Fig 2-1).

Light Interaction With Matter

When light shines on a substance, the light photons are reflected from the surface, transmitted through the substance, absorbed, or scattered by the molecules and particles in the substance.

Reflection

In the study of light reflection by surfaces, there are two limiting cases. The first concerns regular (spectular) reflection from a smooth surface and the second concerns diffuse reflection from a matte surface. In reality, all possible variations are found between these two extremes, for example, reflections from polished wood. The amount of light reflected by a surface is dependent on the intrinsic characteristic of the reflecting surface, the angle of incidence of the light beam, and the refractive indices of the two substances in contact that form the boundary reflective surface.

Transmission

From our daily experience we know that visible light photons are transmitted through colorless glass and water. In such cases, the inci-

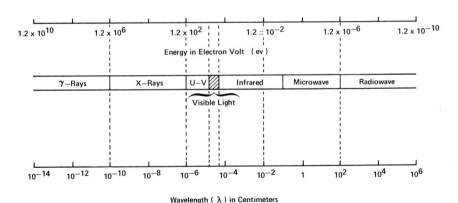

Fig 2–1.—The electromagnetic spectrum: conversion of wavelength to energy is depicted.

dent photons retain their original energies and directions as if they passed through a vacuum. Such a phenomenon does not produce an image. That is why glass doors have to be marked with colored words or pictures to prevent people from walking through them. Images are produced by a combination of selective reflection, scattering, and absorption.

Absorption

A photon that is absorbed could lose its total energy to the absorbing medium (or molecules), with the energy being converted to heat. This is called internal conversion. The requirement for such absorption to occur is the presence of excited energy states in the molecule, where the difference of one higher energy state and the ground state is equal to the incident photon energy. This is studied in the field of spectroscopy where quantum mechanics is used for the calculation of energy states. For example, the oxyhemoglobin molecule has many excited energy states, as illustrated in Figure 2-2. When a photon of 578 nm collides with an oxyhemoglobin molecule at the proper angle, the photon will be absorbed and the oxyhemoglobin molecule will be excited to Excited State I. The energy of the absorbed photon could be converted to heat and then evenly distributed in the molecule and its surroundings, in which case the molecule reverts back to ground state. However, there are alternate pathways. The excited molecule could also lose the extra energy by direct reemission of a photon. This phenomenon includes both fluorescence and phosphorescence depending on the type of excited energy states that can be demonstrated by how soon light is reemitted. A photon is generally reemitted within 10^{-7} seconds in fluorescence and longer than 10^{-5} seconds in phosphorescence.

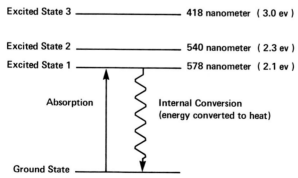

Fig 2–2.—Diagram of electronic energy states of oxyhemoglobin.

Scattering

Photons incident on a substance that are not reflected, transmitted, or absorbed are scattered. There is no rigorous theory of multiple scattering, although many authors have attempted to develop a phenomenological theory of absorption and scattering of tightly packed particle layers. In the majority of the theories, only two constants are introduced, namely, the absorption coefficient and the scattering coefficient. In our discussion of light interaction with matter in transillumination, the system is so complex that we can only discuss it in a qualitative fashion. In scattering interactions, the photon can retain its original energy or lose part of its energy after collision. Elastic collision occurs when the incident photon and scattering particle or molecule do not exchange energy. Such interactions include Rayleigh and Mie scattering. Rayleigh scattering is caused by molecules or particles much smaller than the wavelengths of light ($<0.1\lambda$). The amount of scattering is inversely proportional to the fourth power of the wavelengths, λ^{-4}. This means the shorter wavelengths of light are scattered more severely than the longer wavelengths. For every ten blue waves ($\lambda = 400$ nm) that are scattered, there is only one scattered red wave ($\lambda = 650$ nm). Mie scattering is caused by particles much larger than its wavelength (0.1 to 10λ). It is inversely proportional to wavelength at a range of exponent from 0 to 4 (λ^0 to λ^{-4}).

Inelastic collision occurs when the incident photon loses part of its energy to the scattering particles. The result is a change in photon direction and energy (wavelength). This is called Raman scattering.

All of the above interactions occur between light photons and the organ being transilluminated. The types of interaction that may differentiate between normal and abnormal transillumination images may be attributed to more than two of the above interactions. The first is reflection. Normally, expanded lungs will reflect, absorb, and scatter light in all directions. In a collapsed lung, the pleural surface reflects a major fraction of the transilluminated light. The reflected beams are not scattered significantly by the free air space until they hit the thoracic wall where further scattering by the soft tissues to the external skin surface produces the positive transillumination. In hydrocephalus, the enlarged ventricular wall reflects a considerable amount of light, and, when the cerebrospinal fluid (CSF) is clear, there is less absorption and scattering of the reflected light by the CSF than brain tissue. Again, positive transillumination is produced from the reflected light on the scalp. However, when considerable blood is present in the enlarged ventricle, what should have been a positive transillumination turns negative because of hemoglobin absorption (see Fig 2-2). Absorption, therefore, is the second important light interaction that can affect positive and negative studies.

The optimal application of transillumination has to take into consideration the above factors, and our visual response. Since our vision is only sensitive to the 400- to 700-nm range, with sensitivity dropping off sharply at long wavelengths, any light photon outside this range will have no diagnostic value unless one uses photosensitive detectors that are sensitive beyond the visual range, as applied by Donn et al. (1979). By using a cadmium sulfide photocell, which is sensitive in the range of 350 nm to 750 nm, they were able to detect transilluminated light in the 650-nm to 750-nm range, which is very poorly or not at all detectable by the naked eye.

Another important factor to consider is the strong body tissue absorption at 570 nm down to the ultraviolet light which automatically removes this spectral range from being useful in transillumination as described earlier. Figure 2-3 shows the absorption curves of various

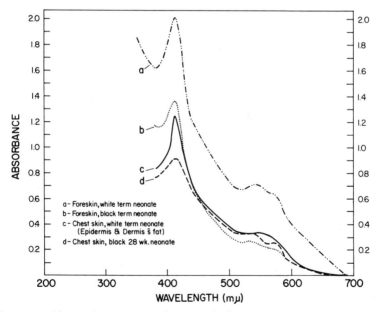

Fig 2–3.—Absorption spectra of neonatal skin specimens in vitro. Relative absorbance on ordinate is measured in log numbers. (From Uy J.O., et al.: Light filtration during transillumination of the neonate: A method to reduce heat buildup in the skin. *Pediatrics* 60:308–312, 1977. Copyright American Academy of Pediatrics 1977. Used by permission.)

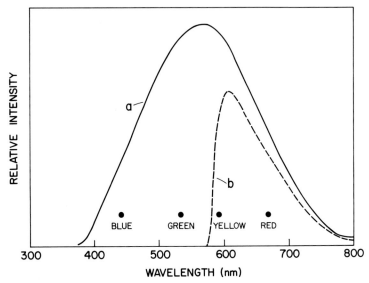

Fig 2–4.—Spectral output of illuminator at its highest output setting without (curve *a*) and with (curve *b*) glass filtration. (From Uy J.O., et al.: Light filtration during transillumination of the neonate: A method to reduce heat buildup in the skin. *Pediatrics* 60:308–312, 1977. Copyright American Academy of Pediatrics 1977. Used by permission.)

body tissues. Uy et al. (1977) demonstrated that when the 400-nm to 570-nm spectral output of the illuminator is filtered out before the light shines on the body, the diagnostic capability of the remaining beam is not compromised (Fig 2-4) and the net result is the favorable reduction of skin heat buildup secondary to photon absorption as demonstrated in Figure 2-5.

In conclusion, the application of transillumination using visual technique is optimized if we use high-intensity light in the range of 550 to 650 nm for determining the presence of pneumothorax or nonhemorrhagic hydrocephalus. If a good, near infrared photodetector is available, and the physician is willing to sacrifice visual acuity, high-intensity light in the range of 500 nm to 800 nm will be adequate for the above cases as well as hemorrhagic hydrocephalus. This latter set-up can overcome the problem of absorption by hemoglobin.

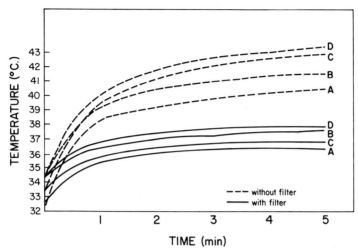

Fig 2–5.—Skin temperature changes in four adult volunteers during forearm transillumination with illuminator at maximum setting. Note marked reduction of temperature rise when light is filtered with orange glass. (From Uy J.O., et al.: Light filtration during transillumination of the neonate: A method to reduce heat buildup in the skin. *Pediatrics* 60:308–312, 1977. Copyright American Academy of Pediatrics 1977. Used by permission.)

REFERENCES

Brown E.B.: *Modern Optics.* Huntington, N.Y., R.E. Kreiger, 1974.

Donn S.M., et al.: Rapid detection of neonatal intracranial hemorrhage by transillumination. *Pediatrics.* 64:843–847, 1979.

Kerker M.: *The Scattering of Light and Other Electromagnetic Radiation.* New York, Academic Press, 1969.

Lim E.C. (ed.): *Excited States.* New York, Academic Press, 1974, vol 1.

Uy J.O., et al.: Light filtration during transillumination of the neonate: A method to reduce heat buildup in the skin. *Pediatrics.* 60:308–312, 1977.

3

Equipment and Principles of Measurement

S.M. Donn, M.D.
B.J. Duchinsky, M.S.

THE EQUIPMENT NECESSARY to perform transillumination can be separated into that required to perform conventional transillumination and that required to perform quantitative transillumination.

Conventional transillumination refers to the traditional use of scattered light in the body. There are three major considerations in conventional transillumination. First, no quantitative record is made of the procedures. Second, there are no standardized techniques for transillumination or detection. Third, only visible light is used. The operator's skill and experience, rather than the equipment, largely determine the success of the technique.

Quantitative transillumination produces a quantitative record of a transillumination procedure, either by recording light images (medical photography) or by making optical measurements (halo size, light intensity, or optical density of tissues). Quantitative transillumination demands standardized techniques and equipment for the light source and detector. Also, the operator is not limited to the visible portion of the spectrum (infrared light can be used).

CONVENTIONAL TRANSILLUMINATION

The most readily available and inexpensive light source is the standard flashlight, powered by two D-cell batteries. Transillumination can be more effectively performed if a good seal can be made between the

23

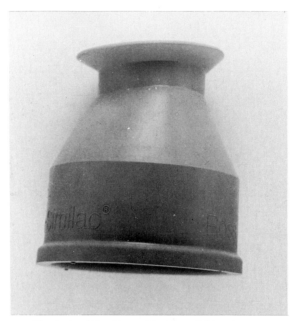

Fig 3–1.—The Trans-Dapter rubber sleeve.

flashlight and skin surface. A rubber sleeve, such as the Trans-Dapter,* is recommended (Fig 3-1). This fits over the illuminating end of the flashlight and acts as a seal to prevent light leakage and permit more accurate assessment (Fig 3-2). The amount of light provided by such a flashlight (in good working order) is generally sufficient to transilluminate the head and large external masses (e.g., cystic hygroma of the neck, sacral meningocele) but is inadequate to detect abnormalities of the thoracic and abdominal cavities.

The Chun Gun† (Fig 3-3) was developed in 1967 by Chun, Cameron, and Voight, and was the first light source designed specifically for pediatric transillumination. It has enabled better standardization of technique and is best suited for transillumination of the skull. It permits the operator to maintain dark adaptation and provides a constant intensity of light over hundreds of examinations. The Chun Gun (Fig 3-4) has a pistol-grip handle and a two-position finger switch. The first

---

*Available free of charge from Ross Laboratories, Columbus, Ohio.

†Radiation Measurements, Inc., P.O. Box 44, Middleton, WI 53562. Approximate cost: $395.

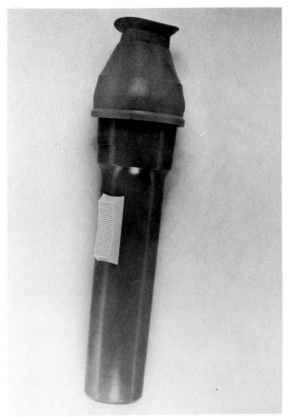

Fig 3–2.—Ordinary flashlight powered by two D-cell batteries, fitted with Trans-Dapter.

position activates a weak red light allowing some ambient lighting without loss of dark adaptation. This allows proper placement of the light probe on the infant. Further depression of the switch activates a 150-watt tungsten projector lamp. This lamp is mounted on the handle, inside a metal cylinder, and is surrounded by large heat fins. A hole is cut in the cylinder, allowing the focused light into a small, half-inch barrel mounted at right angles. There are several glass filters in the barrel. When new, the device has a light output of 5,000 to 10,000 foot-candles (ft-c). In clinical use, the operator places the end of the device against the infant with a light-tight seal. Major drawbacks of this light are its large heat output close to the patient and a power switch that

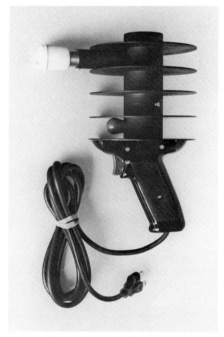

Fig 3–3.—The Chun Gun.

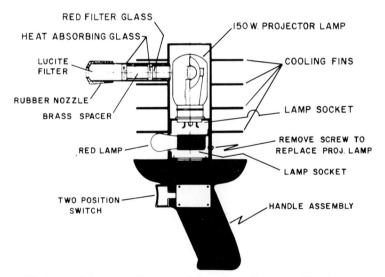

RED FILTER GLASS

HEAT ABSORBING GLASS

150 W. PROJECTOR LAMP

LUCITE FILTER

COOLING FINS

RUBBER NOZZLE

BRASS SPACER

LAMP SOCKET

RED LAMP

REMOVE SCREW TO REPLACE PROJ. LAMP

LAMP SOCKET

TWO POSITION SWITCH

HANDLE ASSEMBLY

Fig 3–4.—Schematic diagram of the Chun Gun transilluminator.

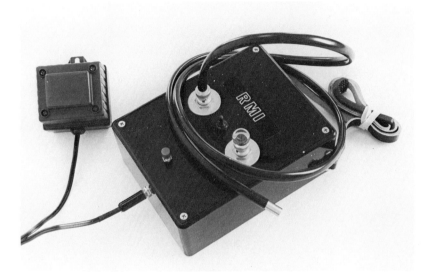

Fig 3–5.—Fiberoptic transilluminator, Model 292, manufactured by Radiation Measurements, Inc., Middleton, WI. It is shown with the 120-V AC power source connected; a portable rechargeable battery pack is also available.

prohibits its use in an oxygen-enriched environment, such as an infant incubator.

The need for a portable, high-intensity light source that could be used throughout the nursery or hospital fostered the development of fiberoptic devices (Fig 3-5). These have two major differences from the Chun Gun. First, the light source, usually a halogen quartz lamp, is separated from the patient by a 3- to 5-foot flexible probe, composed of multiple fiberoptic (light-transmitting) bundles. This eliminates both the heat output and the power switch problems of the Chun Gun. Second, some models are equipped with rheostatically controlled power sources, allowing variability of transillumination from 0 to 12,000 ft-c (before filtration). Table 3-1 compares the features of three commercially available fiberoptic transilluminators.

Surgical illuminators are also in use. These have ultra-high-intensity mercury arc lamps (like those found in 16-mm movie projectors) and fiberoptic bundles to direct the light to a surgical site. The light is much brighter and whiter than that of either a Chun Gun or fiberoptic transilluminator. Provisions are made for beam filtering. Finally, there are some experimental laser transilluminators undergoing investigation.

TABLE 3–1.—FIBEROPTIC LIGHT SOURCES

MODEL	WELCH ALLYN (48300·light with 48210 pipe)	OMNI-SOURCE (NEUROMEDICS, INC.)	RMI MODEL 292
Light source	Halogen 30 watts (Welch Allyn 14V, 04100)	Quartz halogen 200 watts (GE 24V EJL200w)	Quartz halogen 30 watts (GE EKZ 30w 10.8V)
Intensity (ft-c)	4,300 (at 10 cm)	0–2,400 (at 1.75 cm)	4,000–5,000 (at 1.0 cm, est.)
Power source	120V AC	120V AC	120V AC or optional rechargeable Yuasa battery pack
Filtration	In line	Heat and light (may be selected or locked in place)	In line
Weight	9 lb, 10 oz (with stand)	20 lb, 6 oz (with stand)	2 lb (battery pack = 3 lb)
Lamp life	100 hr	80 hr (built-in reserve lamp)	200 hr (built-in reserve lamp)
Approximate cost	$457 (stand = $180)	$1245 (stand = $100)	$495 (battery pack = $150)
Special features	Dissipates heat by conduction (heat sinking; no fan necessary)	Variable intensity, rheostatically controlled	Complete portability with battery pack

Filtering and Safety

As light sources become more powerful, patient safety concerns require beam filtering. Commercial transilluminators use 150- to 300-watt
tungsten or halogen-quartz projector lamps, causing significant problems because of the lamp heat itself, and the patient's exposure to infrared light. To solve the first problem, the lamps are air-cooled, either
by heat fins (free convection, e.g. Chun Gun), cooling fans (forced convection, e.g., Omni-Source), or heat-sinking (conduction, e.g., Welch
Allyn).

Two methods may be used to reduce the considerable amount of
infrared in the light beam. First, dichroic ("cold") mirrors can be used
to shape and filter the beam. These mirrors* have the unique property
of reflecting 90% of the visible light and transmitting 80+% of the infrared light incident on them. Some projector lamps have reflectors made
of dichroic mirrors which pass most of the bulb's infrared light behind
them. Second, special glass infrared filters remove most of the remain-

---

*Edmund Scientific Co., 1976.

ing infrared light before the beam enters the body. Without these filters, high-intensity light sources would be too dangerous to use.

On the Chun Gun an additional safety device was added by force-fitting a 40-mm clear lucite plug in the barrel. The plug provides not only a good degree of protection if the infrared filters are removed, but will also melt and bubble on the end closest to the bulb. This renders the light useless, requiring that it be returned to the factory for correction.

Even with most of the infrared light removed from the beam there were still problems with heat buildup (Kuhns et al., 1976) and occasionally thermal injury (Wyman, 1978; Church and Adamkin, 1981). Uy and associates (1977) found that tissue converts shorter visible wavelengths (blue and green light) into heat (see chap. 2). Light escaping from the body during transillumination is yellow to red in color, suggesting that blue and green light are absorbed. Consequently, most light sources now have red Corning glass filters that eliminate the blue-green light. The reddish-orange light does not appear to cause major problems for operators (except possibly for those with red-green color blindness).

QUANTITATIVE TRANSILLUMINATION

Quantitative transillumination uses standard techniques to record a transillumination procedure, either by storing the image or by making optical measurements. Difficult problems arise with quantitating transillumination if one tries to avoid burdening conventional transillumination with complex procedures and expensive equipment.

Generally speaking, quantitative transillumination involves seven elements, six of which have controllable variables (tissue excluded). The key is in trying to control all the variables for an optimum perceptible output. These six elements are as follows:

1. *Light source.* The light intensity and spectrum are the most important qualities of the light source. Intensity is the easiest to change and, consequently, the hardest to standardize. There are intensity boundaries, however. Too dim a source can put measurements out of the sensor's range, while too bright a source tends to "wash out" results as loud background noise (light corona) masks the useful signals.

Light intensity is closely related to light spectrum. The light spectrum limits intensity when it contains heat-generating radiation, such as the shorter blue-green wavelengths or the longer near-infrared wavelengths. The light spectrum can be modified with filters.

2. *Sensor.* The sensor's function is to convert the transilluminated

light into electrical energy or to use it to divert chemical reactions. There are a wide variety of sensors to choose from: eyes, camera, and film, and a host of photodetectors. Two important sensor characteristics are sensitivity and spectral response. Together, they are used to select the information that will eventually be displayed. Temperature, pressure, or electrical potentials are not sensed here, since no one as yet has reported a measurable physiologic change during transillumination.

3. *Signal processing.* Except in the brain, signal processing is limited to developing film or manipulating electric signals. Electronic signal processing is usually amplification and analog-to-digital conversion of DC signals, although pulsed source-sensor systems also require sample-and-hold and peak detection circuits.

4. *Output display.* Output displays fall into the same two categories as the sensor and signal processing, namely, medical images and optical measurements. Common output displays are camera film and analog or digital panel meters.

5. *Data storage.* Like the output display, data storage depends on the sensor and signal processing. Common data storage methods are memory, camera film, and manual records. Digital information is not stored electronically.

6. *Control and feedback.* Control and feedback "fine tune" the entire system during transillumination. They take many forms: adjusting the light source's intensity or filtering, manipulating the patient, changing the senor's sensitivity or position, changing the type of camera film, or adjusting the scale of an electronic meter.

Methods

There are three methods of quantitating transillumination. They differ in how closely they relate to conventional transillumination.

In the first method, quantitative transillumination supplements conventional procedures. Known as *first-generation systems*, these systems differ from the other two by allowing a physician to use conventional transillumination as before and quantitate the results. Previous work and current research center on two approaches: medical photography and optical measurements. First-generation systems are the easiest for researchers to design and test, and for physicians to accept.

Second-generation systems do not use conventional transilluminators. These systems use infrared light sources and there is nothing for the clinician to "see" during transillumination. Second-generation transilluminators are photoplethysmographs—instruments that measure "optical impedance" of tissues. Previous work and current research center on clinical psychological transducers, pulsed cranial transilluminators, and matched infrared emitter-detector pairs.

A third method is even further removed from conventional transillumination. Here, the transilluminator would be used as a stimulator and the physician would measure any physiologic change during transillumination. Since there has been no research published in this area, this method cannot be further discussed.

First-Generation Systems: Previous Work

A technique for producing a permanent radiographic record of transillumination was described by Martin et al. in 1977. This method has utilized photography with a 35-mm single lens reflex camera and Kodak Plus-X film (any film that can be processed in the automatic x-ray processor may be substituted). Photographs are taken in a dimly lit room, at the widest possible aperture (generally f/1.4–2.0) for ⅛ to 1 second. The transillumination is initially performed in a completely darkened room, so that the abnormal finding is located. Room lighting is then gradually increased until the finding is barely discernible to the non-dark-adapted eye. The transilluminated structure may be photographed, then the film processed in the regular 90-second x-ray processor. Negatives can be enlarged and printed on Kodak RPM mammography film rather than paper, yielding a transparent end-product which can be made part of the patient's x-ray folder.

CORONA MEASUREMENTS.—One problem with conventional transillumination is establishing norms for infants without abnormalities that easily "light up." The corona or halo surrounding the transilluminator tip contains the only diagnostic information. Three studies have been published using a Chun Gun for establishing cranial transilluminator norms. Cheldelin et al. (1975) made measurements of corona size using a circumferential ruler attached to the Chun Gun tip. Vyhmeister et al. (1977) studied infants with a clear, flexible, graduated disk attached to the tip. Finally, Swick et al. (1976) had a more complicated procedure using calipers and a tape measure laid on the child's head.

First-Generation Systems: Current Research

PHOTODETECTORS.—Several photodetectors are suitable for quantitative transillumination. Photoconductive cells (CdS photoresistors) provide medium sensitivity at a low cost. The cells can produce signals with light levels as low as 0.0001 ft-c, and come in a variety of spectral responses. One of the more undesirable characteristics of photoconductive cells is their "memory," a hysteresis-like effect in their illumination vs. resistance curve due to the illumination level at which the cell is stored. This can cause instabilities, especially at low light levels. Another nuisance is the very long time constants at very low light levels. Extremely large cell resistances are possible at these levels.

Photodiodes are silicon PN junction diodes whose current under-reverse bias is a function of illumination. Response times are on the order of nanoseconds. Their spectral response peaks symmetrically at 850–900 nm (near-infrared). Photodiodes are inherently stable devices. They can also act as current generators without bias under very bright illumination.

Phototransistors are essentially transistors with the light-generated base current multiplied by the transistor current gain. Photosensitivity to a given light level can be 100 to 500 times larger than for a photodiode. Speed and spectral response are comparable to photodiodes. A photo-darlington is a phototransistor cascaded with a second transistor for further current gain. These devices are ideal for measuring extremely low light levels.

Second-Generation Systems: Previous Work

PSYCHOPHYSIOLOGIC TRANSDUCERS.—Psychophysiologists rely on photoplethysmography to measure relative changes in peripheral vascular activity. This technique uses a small light source and photodetector attached to a recording site like a finger or earlobe. Changes in light intensity seen by the sensor are related to vascular changes in the underlying tissue.

In the past, miniature tungsten lamps and photoresistors were used, with all their inherent problems. Sensor Technology, Inc., manufactures a device containing both an infrared LED and phototransistor in the same package (STRT-850A). This marks the advent of the second-generation system. However, practical applications to neonatology and pediatrics are difficult because of the low output of the infrared LED.

PULSED TRANSILLUMINATORS.—These devices have combined photoplethysmography with pediatric transillumination. Johnson and colleagues (1973) designed a cranial transilluminator using a gallium arsenide infrared LED and a silicon phototransistor spaced three centimeters apart. An oscillator triggers a 15-ampere pulse of the LED and activates a sample-and-hold circuit to read the phototransistor's peak pulse height. Pulsing the LED produces intense bursts of infrared light without the danger of heating tissue or destroying the LED, as with continuous illumination.

Physio-Control Corp. built and tested two prototypes of Johnson's pulsed cranial transilluminator (Hayden et al., 1975). This meter was calibrated to read the transmitted infrared intensity in optical density units per centimeter, OD/cm. Areas filled with clear fluid would absorb less infrared light and give lower optical density readings.

Although the device was an overall success, based on 222 infants, Physio-Control Corp. did not pursue the matter further.

Light Meters

Two light meters, both manufactured by Radiation Measurements, Inc., Middleton, WI, may prove useful to those who practice transillumination.

The first of these, Model 294A (Fig 3-6), is a photodiode light meter, requiring no external power. We recommend that this device be used on a regular basis to monitor the output of fiberoptic transilluminators. We have previously reported the eventual breakage of fiberoptic bundles with subsequent loss of light intensity (Fig 3-7) (Donn et al., 1980). Periodic measurement of light output, which is displayed on the meter in microamperes, will alert the user to fiberoptic or bulb malfunction.

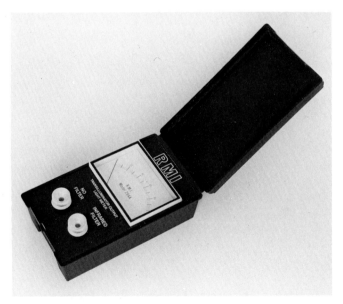

Fig 3–6.—Transillumination output light meter, Model 294A, manufactured by Radiation Measurements, Inc., Middleton, WI.

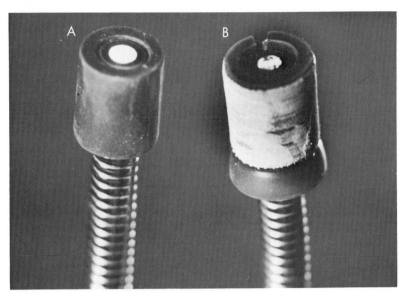

Fig 3–7.—Comparison of two identical fiberoptic light probes. Probe *A* is new. Probe *B* is older and shows loss of light transmission through breakage of fiberoptic fibers (dark areas). It has only 20% of the intensity of probe *A*. (From Donn S.M., et al.: Transillumination—a technical note. *Pediatrics* 66:813–814, 1980. Copyright American Academy of Pediatrics 1980. Used by permission.)

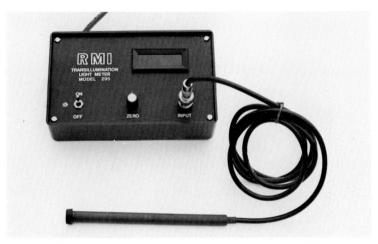

Fig 3–8.—Transillumination light meter, Model 295.

The meter also enables standardization of two or more light sources. It costs about $75.

The other meter, Model TLM295 (Fig 3-8), has proved useful for quantitative transillumination. This device is a photodiode detector which detects light in the 400- to 650-nm range. The intensity of light is displayed on a digital screen and the units correspond to a range of 10^{-3} to 10^{-2} ft-c. The device requires external power for operation, though the actual current passing through the photocell is only 10^{-4} to 10^{-2} milliamps. The light detection probe is flexible and may be placed comfortably against skin surfaces. Thus far a similar meter using a cadmium sulfide photocell has only been applied to quantitative cranial transillumination (Donn et al., 1979). However, it appears to have great potential and may enable subtle changes in transillumination and even earlier detection of pneumothorax, pneumomediastinum, or pneumoperitoneum.

REFERENCES

Cheldelin L.V., et al.: Normal values for transillumination of skull using a new light source. *J. Pediatr.* 87:937–938, 1975.

Church S., Adamkin D.H.: Transillumination in neonatal intensive care: A possible iatrogenic complication. *South. Med. J.* 74:76–77, 1981.

Donn S.M., et al.: Rapid detection of neonatal intracranial hemorrhage by transillumination. *Pediatrics* 64:843–847, 1979.

Donn S.M., et al.: Transillumination—a technical note. *Pediatrics* 66:813–814, 1980.

Hayden P.W., et al.: A pulsed transilluminator for the infant cranium. *Clin. Pediatr.* 14:627–632, 1975.

Information and instruction sheet: Cold mirror. Edmund Scientific Co. 42:414, 1976.

Johnson C.C., et al.: Infant cranial transillumination. *Med. Instrum.* 7:62, 1973.

Kuhns L.R., et al.: A caution about using photoillumination devices. *Pediatrics* 57:975–976, 1976.

Martin A.J., et al.: Production of a permanent radiographic record of transillumination of the neonate. *Radiology* 122:540–541, 1977.

Swick H.M., et al.: Transillumination of the skull in premature infants. *Pediatrics* 58:658–664, 1976.

Uy J.O., et al.: Light filtration during transillumination of the neonate: A method to reduce heat buildup in the skin. *Pediatrics* 60:308–312, 1977.

Vyhmeister N., et al.: Cranial transillumination norms of the premature infant. *J. Pediatr.* 91:980–982, 1977.

Wyman M.L.: Uses of transillumination in the newborn nursery. *Perinatol./Neonatol.* Jan./Feb. 1978.

Part II

CLINICAL TRANSILLUMINATION

S. M. Donn, M.D.
L. R. Kuhns, M.D.

4

General Techniques of Transillumination

USE OF A VERY BRIGHT light source in clinical transillumination increases the accuracy of the technique. A lamp that produces 3,000 to 5,000 foot-candles is generally required to transilluminate accurately most structures, even in neonates. When this lamp source is filtered, the heat buildup in the skin and subcutaneous tissues becomes minimal (see chap. 2). What had been a problem in the past, the transmission of light to the neonate or young infant, has now been eased with the fiberoptic or gel probe transmission of light. A flexible or semiflexible fiberoptic probe can bring the light to the neonate even in an incubator. The probe tip can be used much as an examining finger and placed in many areas. A rubber cuff is generally required around the light probe tip so that the corona of light that occurs around the probe tip in the subcutaneous fat is masked. This allows the examiner to look at the area with better dark adaptation.

With very bright light sources, minimal dark adaptation is necessary, particularly if the room can be made completely dark or dimmed considerably. The examiner then approaches the mass or suspected mass from several different directions. In some instances, a given direction is best and this can be predicted. For example, for kidney transillumination, the probe tip should be placed in the upper quadrant, pushed deep into the abdomen, and one should look at the costovertebral angle on that side for abnormal kidney transillumination. One should try to rotate the patient into several positions which allow bowel loops to float away from the probe tip so as to determine that a mass is being transilluminated rather than a bowel loop. The probe tip should be used very gently.

With adequate filtration so that heat buildup is reduced, there is no theoretical limit to the length of time which the probe tip can be applied to any one area. However, it is wise to limit the use of the probe to any one area to approximately 15 to 20 seconds, so the probe tip itself will not mechanically irritate the skin. Heat buildup is not a danger when adequate filtration is used (Uy et al., 1977). The probe tip is then gently withdrawn and is reinserted and directed in a slightly different direction. This allows one to examine the entire area for abnormal transillumination. Often only one angle produces the best view of the transilluminating structure.

The child must be cooperative or adequately immobilized. For adequate abdominal transillumination the child must be able to relax the abdomen. For thoracic transillumination or head transillumination in the neonate, immobilization is usually not required. The probe tip can easily be placed on the head or the chest and the young infant or neonate will not move significantly, so that adequate transillumination is possible. One should always examine both sides of the chest, abdomen, or head and compare the transillumination from each. It is often possible then to compare a relatively normal side with an abnormal side. Transmission transillumination is possible in the extremities and in the kidney areas. In most other areas, the probe tip is applied to the region and reflected transillumination is evaluated.

COMPARISON WITH OTHER DIAGNOSTIC IMAGING TECHNIQUES

Transillumination is most aptly compared to ultrasonography. Both techniques are relatively harmless because they employ no ionizing radiation, and both have been touted as being very good in differentiating fluid-filled from solid structures. One of the major differences between transillumination and ultrasound is that transillumination produces a transmission and/or reflection view of the entire region of interest and delineates air- or fluid-filled structures in relation to the entire region. Ultrasound produces cross-sectional images which must be pieced together in the observer's mind in order to understand the entire three-dimensional outline of a mass or organ. It is much easier for the observer to understand anatomical relationships with transillumination.

The major disadvantage of transillumination, as compared to ultrasound, is that it is difficult to obtain hard copy. Photography with very high-speed color film will produce a permanent record of the transillumination, but it is difficult to obtain just the right exposure for hard copy. On the other hand, ultrasound technology has advanced to a state where it is extremely easy to make permanent hard copy or videotape records of the ultrasound images. The accuracy of ultrasound and transillumination is probably about equal when applied to the neonate. In the older child, as the abdominal wall becomes thicker and the subcutaneous fat increases, transillumination becomes less and less reliable. Ultrasonography, however, is an excellent diagnostic technique in cooperative children of any age.

While respiratory motion can affect the findings of ultrasonography, since an organ or structure can move into and out of the sections being scanned, respiratory variation has little effect on the use of transillumination. A moving structure is easily transilluminated and the structure can be seen through the abdominal or chest wall even if respiratory motion occurs.

Ultrasonography characterizes a mass or structure as being sonolucent or echogenic. Sonolucent is somewhat equivalent to being fluid-filled, though not all the time. Some very uniform tumors with little fibrous tissues, such as lymphoma, and some collections, such as hematomas or abscesses, can be completely sonolucent on ultrasonography during certain stages of their evolution. These structures can be diagnosed by ultrasonography as cystic when they are not. On the other hand, when transillumination produces a bright glow from a structure, the structure is either air-filled or fluid-filled, and there is no question about this. Very few solid structures will transilluminate, no matter how uniform the cellular structure and how lacking it is in fibrous tissue. Fat-filled structures transilluminate much less intensely than air- or fluid-filled structures. In this respect, transillumination is somewhat more reliable than ultrasonography when applied to the neonate. For example, soon after an intraventricular hemorrhage in the neonate the ventricles can be completely sonolucent on ultrasonography, but during transillumination the blood in the ventricles allows little or no passage of light, thus indicating the presence of a bleed. Gas-filled structures interposed between a mass and the skin surface will prevent successful ultrasonography of that mass.

Comparison of transillumination with other diagnostic imaging techniques is less applicable. Almost all other imaging techniques require ionizing radiation. The simplest comparison is between transillumination and routine radiography. A radiograph of the abdomen, for example, is quite helpful when used in conjunction with transillumination. If a mass is detected which does transilluminate abnormally, it may be filled with air or fluid. A simple abdominal radiograph will settle the question as to whether the mass is fluid-filled or air-containing. Since routine radiographs require very little radiation, it is certainly helpful in many circumstances to obtain a radiograph and perform transillumination at the same time. An alternative solution would be to perform ultrasonography at the same time as transillumination, but in many instances ultrasound is not as available as routine radiography.

Computed tomography can also be employed as a cross-sectional technique for delineating masses and helping to evaluate whether a mass is cystic or solid. Computerized tomograms require much more radiation than routine radiographs and are thus less competitive with transillumination than are ultrasonography and radiography. The physical density of a structure is delineated by computerized tomography. If the physical density of the structure is that of water, then it can be assumed that the structure is fluid-filled. However, some tumors that become necrotic and are actually filled with necrotic debris have a central density which is equivalent to that of water. They are not in a true sense cystic and are not benign. Transillumination is somewhat more reliable in determining whether a mass is cystic or solid and in suggesting whether it is benign or malignant when compared with computed tomography. Angiography, which has been classically performed by placing a catheter through the femoral artery and into the aorta and then directing the tip into selected vessels, is used less frequently in children today because it places the femoral artery at risk. The amount of radiation from angiography is considerably more than that from radiography, which makes angiography not very competitive with transillumination.

Thermography, which consists of measuring the infrared irradiation occurring from internal organs through the subcutaneous tissues, is often complementary to transillumination. Thermography gives some indication as to the vascular perfusion of an organ or mass. An organ or mass with a great deal of blood flow will appear hot on the thermogram because of its heat emission through the abdominal or chest wall, whereas a cystic or necrotic mass with little blood flow will appear cold in relation to surrounding structures. Thermography, which requires no ionizing radiation, has not been used to a great extent in pediatric practice and probably should be utilized more. We have found that thermography is often complementary to transillumination in delineating whether a lesion is hypervascular or not, which is some indication as to whether the mass may be malignant.

Radioisotope imaging is also employed. A minimal to moderate amount of radiation is involved depending on the imaging technique. Dynamic studies can be performed with radioisotopes which allow assessment of physiologic functions and vascular perfusion. The use of radioisotopes to delineate renal function and/or obstruction is very useful and this is often more of a diagnostic aid than is transillumination. However, a mass with lack of accumulation of radioactivity on the radioisotope scan can result from either a necrotic tumor or a cystic structure; here, transillumination is more accurate than the radioisotope scan in delineating the true nature of a lesion.

REFERENCE

Uy J.O., et al.: Light filtration during transillumination of the neonate: A method to reduce heat buildup in the skin. *Pediatrics* 60:308–312, 1977.

5

Transillumination of the Head and Neck

THE HEAD

Transillumination of the head should be considered a standard part of the newborn neurologic examination. It is an inexpensive, noninvasive, simple test which may give valuable clues to several developmental brain anomalies and acquired lesions. Elaborate equipment is not necessary; a standard battery-powered flashlight with a rubber sleeve (e.g., the "Trans-Dapter") around the light rim will generally suffice, but, for optimal results, it is best to use the same light sources as those for chest transillumination.

Technique

The infant should be examined in as dark a room as possible. If a battery-powered flashlight is used, the examiner should allow adequate time for dark adaptation. The infant should be held in an upright or sitting position. The light source is applied to the infant's head. A good seal is achieved when only a small rim of transillumination (corona) can be seen around the edge of the light source when it is pressed against the skull. The light source is initially placed over the anterior fontanelle (Fig 5-1), then moved laterally along the coronal suture to the ears (Fig 5-2), then to the frontoparietal regions of each side (Figs 5-3, 5-4). The infant is then turned so that the posterior skull may be transilluminated in the same manner (Fig 5-5), from the base to the ears laterally, and the anterior fontanelle anteriorly. Careful observation of the degree of lucency is made in each position.

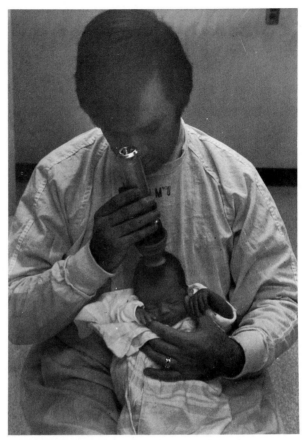

Fig 5–1.—Transillumination of the infant's head. Light source is initially applied over the anterior fontanelle.

Normal Transillumination

Many factors affect the degree of light transmission, especially gestational age and extracranial and intracranial features. Since prematurity is associated with increased brain water content, thinner cranial bones, and decreased scalp thickness, the degree of transillumination is inversely proportional to gestational age. The degree of transillumination (assessed by the size of the corona) is normally not uniform over the skull; the frontal region generally displays the greatest corona, fol-

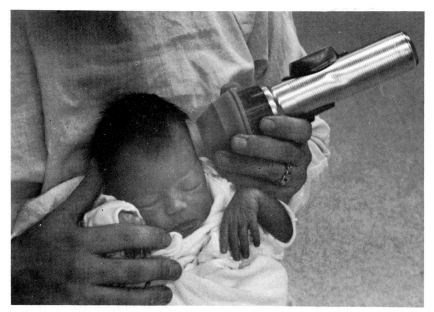

Fig 5–2.—Transillumination of the infant's head. Light source placed over coronal suture just above the ear.

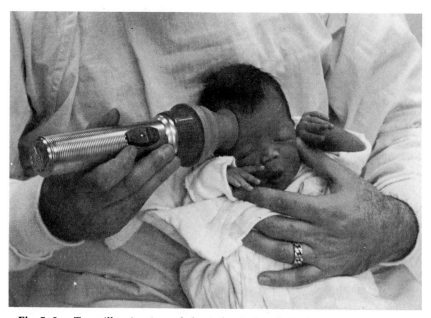

Fig 5–3.—Transillumination of the infant's head. Light source placed over fronto-parietal region.

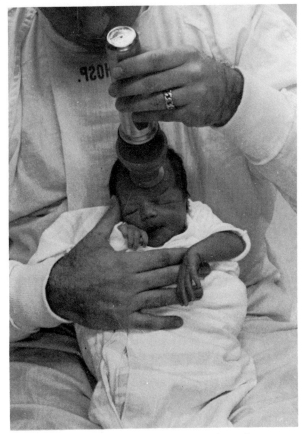

Fig 5–4.—Transillumination of the infant's head. Light source placed over the frontal region.

lowed closely by the parietal region. The entire frontal region may light up and still contain a normal brain.

Extracranial factors may increase or decrease transillumination. Those factors tending to increase transillumination include a thin skull, edema (e.g., caput succedaneum) or increased subcutaneous fat in the scalp, lightly pigmented skin, sparse or blonde hair, and fluid collections (other than blood) between the light and the skull. Factors tending to decrease transillumination include a thick skull, bloody or turbid fluid collections, thick dark hair, and pigmented skin. Many of these differences can be lessened if the intensity of the light source is increased

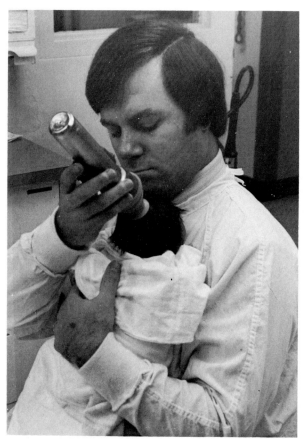

Fig 5–5.—Transillumination of the infant's head. Light source placed over the occipital (posterior) region.

(Volpe, 1981). For this reason we prefer the Chun Gun to an ordinary flashlight; however, if the intensity is too great (e.g., a fiberoptic light source), it becomes difficult to differentiate normal from abnormal.

An elaborate investigation of normal values for cranial transillumination was performed by Vyhmeister, Schneider, and Cha (1977), using the Chun Gun, in which they measured the radius of the maximal corona in the frontal, parietal, and occipital positions in 95 observations of infants of gestational ages from 26 to 42 weeks. Figure 5-6 shows their data and indicates decreasing frontal and parietal transillumination with increasing gestational age, while occipital transillumination

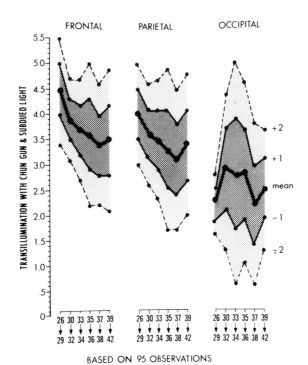

BASED ON 95 OBSERVATIONS

Fig 5–6.—Transillumination of the premature infant. Combined study of all infants measured at birth or at varying ages in weeks. Transillumination measurements are the radius in centimeters of the maximal halo of light from the center of the light source (Chun Gun). Only important variable was the amount of hair, while infant's sex, right and left hemispheres, skin, and hair color were not found to be significant. Standard deviations are given in dotted areas. (From Vyhmeister N., et al.: Cranial transillumination norms of the premature infant. *J. Pediatr.* 91:980–982, 1977. Used by permission.)

was more variable. Their data also suggest a potential use of transillumination in delineating normal head growth and "catch-up" head growth from central nervous system anomalies and hydrocephalus.

Abnormal Transillumination

Abnormal transillumination may result from intracranial factors which increase or decrease light transmission. Collections of fluid in the subdural or subarachnoid spaces, or parenchyma will increase transillumination, as will decreased or thin cerebral mantle. Collections of blood, which absorb light, will decrease transillumination (Volpe, 1981). Each of these conditions is discussed below.

Hydranencephaly

Hydranencephaly is a condition in which there is a virtual absence of the telencephalon in the distribution of the carotid arteries. If cortical tissue is present, there is generally a large cystic cavity surrounded by a meningeal covering, often accompanied by small islands of cortex and a gliotic layer. This condition has also been reported to occur, although rarely, in the distribution of the vertebral-basilar system, in which case the cerebellum is replaced by a thin membrane which adheres to the dura, and is associated with other congenital anomalies (Roessmann and Parks, 1978).

Transillumination of the skull of an infant with hydranencephaly is diagnostic. The procedure demonstrates grossly abnormal transillumination, with markedly increased lucency in all areas above the posterior fossa; the entire anterior and middle cranial fossae show this pattern. A dark structure running along the midline posteriorly to the torcula may be noted; this is the sagittal sinus. (This may also be identified in preterm infants normally.) The transillumination is so intense that the light may be observed to shine through the pupils. Transillumination tends to normalize more posteriorly, beneath the tentorium cerebelli (Haller, 1981).

Hydrocephalus

Hydrocephalus may be congenital, as in congenital aqueductal stenosis or in Arnold-Chiari malformation, or acquired, as when it follows intracranial hemorrhage or infection.

In the immediate newborn period it may be difficult to diagnose hydrocephalus by transillumination until the cerebral cortex has been compressed to less than 1.0 cm in thickness (Volpe, 1981). Conditions resulting in hydrocephalus in the neonatal period tend to be symmetric, and abnormally increased lucency is seen bilaterally in a supratentorial location, generally in the posterior parietal region. Most likely this represents ventriculomegaly with dilation of the occipital horns of the lateral ventricles and increased cerebrospinal fluid content causing the increase in light transmission (color plate I).

Porencephaly

Porencephalic cysts contain cerebrospinal fluid but are not lined with ependyma and have no choroidal tissue. Cysts may be singular or multiple. Their origin may be related to schizencephaly (failure of sulcation and migration) or focal cerebral destruction (encephaloclastic cysts). They may communicate either internally with the ventricular system, or externally with the subarachnoid space, though this is rare. They may be seen in association with hydrocephalus and may be expansile. Large cysts are common and these may occupy the entire space from the ependyma to the meninges.

Upon transillumination increased lucency is likely to occur if the underlying cerebral mantle is less than 1.0 cm thick (as in hydrocephalus). The cysts tend to be fairly well circumscribed and may resemble simple subarachnoid cysts cephalad to the posterior fossa.

The value of cranial transillumination in the diagnosis of congenital porencephaly was demonstrated by Nixon et al. in a series of 18 patients. Nine of 10 patients with unilateral porencephalic cysts transilluminated positively. Three of 5 patients with bilateral cysts also had positive transilluminations, and there was a high degree of correlation between the location of the cysts on transillumination and radiographic studies. Some of the cases showed a shift of the sagittal sinus from the midline on transillumination toward the side with the cyst (Nixon et al., 1974).

Dandy-Walker Syndrome

In this syndrome, the foramina of Magendie and Luschka are congenitally obstructed; as a result, a large fluid-filled cyst develops which is continuous with the fourth ventricle. Cerebellar hypoplasia is also associated with this syndrome, and a variant form may have absence of the vermis with normal cerebellar hemispheres.

The abnormal appearance of such a cyst on transillumination is limited to the posterior fossa, usually in the midline. Transillumination above the tentorium cerebelli appears normal. Dandy-Walker cysts are usually triangular in shape and show circumscribed lateral margins. Transillumination demonstrates the abnormally located attachment of the tentorium cerebelli and within it the massively enlarged fourth ventricle (Haller, 1981).

Posterior Fossa Arachnoidal Cysts

As with the Dandy-Walker syndrome, the abnormal transillumination is limited to the infratentorial region. However, arachnoidal cysts display a lobulated pattern rather than a sharply demarcated one and the uppermost attachment of tentorium is seen as the peak of the lobulation. The irregularly transilluminated area corresponds to the cyst (Figs 5-7, 5-8, 5-9;

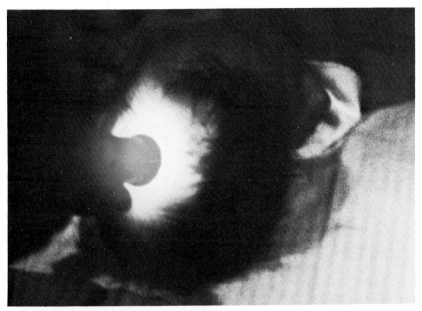

Fig 5–7.—Transillumination of the head of an infant with congenital macrocephaly secondary to a posterior fossa arachnoidal cyst. Note the lobulated pattern of lucency; at the peak of lucency is the attachment of the tentorium.

color plate II). The cerebellum is normal in this anomaly, though it may be deformed or displaced by a large cyst (Haller, 1981).

Subdural Effusion

Subdural effusions are generally associated with infections (meningitis) or old subdural hematomas after lysis of red blood cells. Accumulation of fluid in the subdural space increases transillumination above the tentorium. The condition may be either unilateral or bilateral and discernible by transillumination. The abnormally transilluminated area is adjacent to the sagittal sinus, which may be seen as a midline shadow along the medial border of the effusion. The area of lucency may extend to the parietal region posteriorly or to the frontal region anteriorly (Haller, 1981).

Subdural effusions can be differentiated from increased fluid in the subarachnoid space secondary to cerebral atrophy. In the latter condition there is also abnormally increased transillumination, but the bor-

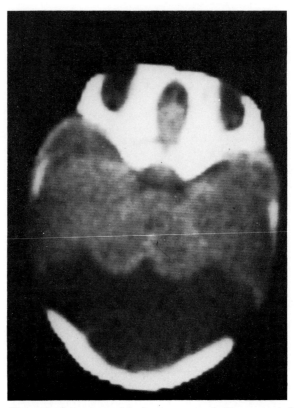

Fig 5–8.—Computed tomographic brain scan of the same infant demonstrates a dilated cystic structure in the posterior fossa.

der of the lucent area is irregular in pattern. With subdural effusion, the border is smooth. In addition, subdural effusions may be differentiated by increased transillumination from scalp edema. With scalp edema, the lucent area may cross the midline, not appear medially confined by the sagittal sinus, and is increased in dependent portions of the head (Haller, 1981).

Subdural Hematoma

In contrast to subdural effusions, subdural hematomas result in markedly decreased transillumination in the acute stages, as light is absorbed by blood. As the character of the fluid changes from grossly hemorrhagic to xanthochromic, light transmission appears and transil-

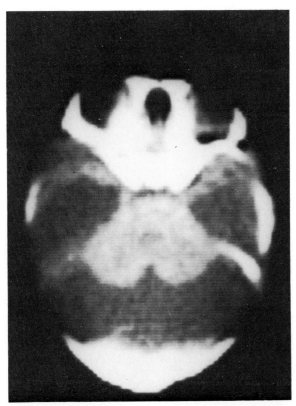

Fig 5–9.—Computed tomographic brain scan of the same infant following intrathecal metrizamide injection. This demonstrated that the cyst did not communicate with the fourth ventricle and ruled out a Dandy-Walker malformation.

lumination returns to normal, then increases. Decreased transillumination is also observed in other conditions resulting in localized hemorrhage, such as cephalhematoma and subgaleal hematoma. In these conditions, an associated subdural hematoma cannot be excluded by transillumination.

Skull Fracture

A rare complication which may follow diastatic linear skull fractures in very young children is the development of herniation of cranial contents and subsequent expansion of the fracture. We applied transillu-

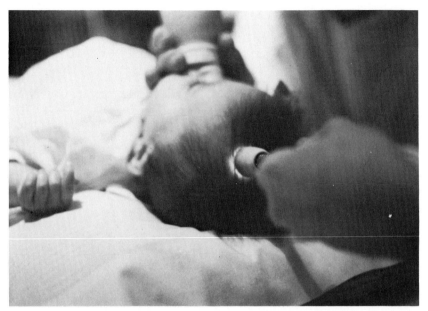

Fig 5–10.—Probe tip of transilluminating light is placed slightly to left of anterior fontanelle. Narrow corona of light is seen around probe tip. (From Kuhns L.R., et al.: Transillumination detection of a growing skull fracture. *Am. J. Dis. Child.* 131:889–892, 1977. Copyright 1977, American Medical Association. Used by permission.)

mination to an 8-month-old infant following a linear skull fracture which occurred two months earlier. We demonstrated an area of lucency in the right frontoparietal region (Figs 5-10, 5-11) and follow-up roentgenograms of the skull displayed enlargement of the original fracture (Fig 5-12). Computed tomographic brain scanning was then performed and showed protruding cerebral cortical tissue. At surgery, contused cerebrum was seen herniating through a dural defect (Kuhns et al., 1977). With a fracture of this sort, brain porencephalic cysts, and arachnoid cysts have all been reported to occur, protruding through the fracture line, and extending the fracture. Transillumination on a frequent basis can aid in the early diagnosis and treatment of this condition. Because it is nonionizing, noninvasive, and inexpensive, routine serial transillumination should be utilized in this situation. It is essential that the entire skull be transilluminated since herniation may also occur through the sutures as well as the defect.

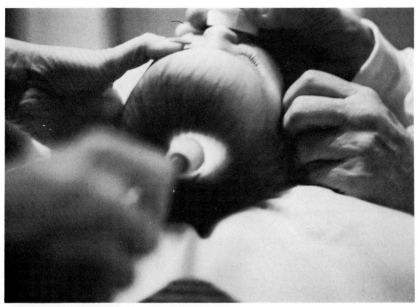

Fig 5–11.—Probe tip placed just to right of anterior fontanelle. Large area transilluminates to right of probe tip. As probe tip was moved toward patient's right ear, area of abnormal transillumination was noted to extend toward right occiput. (From Kuhns L.R., et al.: Transillumination detection of a growing skull fracture. *Am. J. Dis. Child.* 131:889–892, 1977. Copyright 1977, American Medical Association. Used by permission.)

Quantitative Cranial Transillumination

Application of both simple and sophisticated biophysical devices has enabled quantification of transillumination. These devices utilize the principles of light absorption and allow a more objective measurement of transillumination.

Pulsed Transillumination

Hayden et al. (1975) described the use of a pulsed transilluminator of the infant cranium and its use in the detection of abnormal patterns of transillumination. This device consists of a light emitter and a light detector combined into a single hand-held unit which is applied to the cranium. The light source is an infrared-emitting gallium arsenide diode. Light is detected by a silicon photodetector diode, placed 3 cm from the light source. An oscillating 15-amp pulse is delivered to the emitter

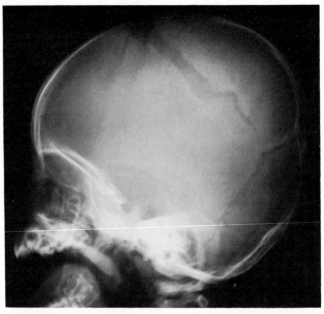

Fig 5–12.—Right lateral skull roentgenogram at time of transillumination. Size of original parietal skull fracture is noted just anterior to lambdoid suture. Growing skull fracture is noted more anteriorly. (From Kuhns L.R., et al.: Transillumination detection of a growing skull fracture. *Am. J. Dis. Child.* 131:889–892, 1977. Copyright 1977, American Medical Association. Used by permission.)

and the peak pulse height is recorded by a sample-hold circuit. The intensity of the transmitted infrared light is read by the light detector and is recorded as optical density units per centimeter (OD/cm). Thus, areas of increased transillumination (e.g., fluid-filled cysts) will give lower OD because of less light absorbance than will areas of decreased transillumination (e.g., blood-filled spaces) because of greater absorbance of light.

Hayden and associates transilluminated 160 normal-term infants and found that the occipital region was invariably 0.1 OD/cm greater than the frontal area. Frontal area OD ranged from 1.2 to 1.9. Readings were also symmetric with respect to corresponding left and right sides. Sixty-two preterm infants were transilluminated, and found to have a mean OD reading of 1.46 (1.2–1.8). Greater transillumination showed a correlation with decreasing gestational age. Skin pigmentation (in seven black babies) increased OD readings by 0.1–0.2 units compared to white babies, but the other relationships (e.g., frontal-occipital, left-right) still prevailed.

Fifty-nine infants suspected of having intracranial pathology were screened by this technique (ages newborn to 5 years). Among the conditions showing abnormal OD were caput succedaneum (2), cephalhematoma (2), hydrocephalus (12), intracerebral cysts (4), acute subdural hematoma (1), postinfectious effusions (2), cerebral atrophy (3), and frontal prominence with microtia (1). Abnormal conditions which showed age-appropriate OD were microcephaly (5), familial cephalomegaly (3), suture diastasis secondary to brain tumor (1), and asymmetric skull (Beal's syndrome) (1). Additionally, 10 preterm infants showed an OD lower than that at term, which also increased with age.

The investigators point out that it is essential to transilluminate the *entire* cranium in order to detect significant patterns of transillumination. The actual OD measurements may be within normal limits in a child with hydrocephalus, but there will be a loss of the normal frontal-greater-than-occipital pattern. The authors also emphasize the primary usefulness of the technique as a screening device, indicating which infants may need more sophisticated diagnostic evaluations. (Unfortunately, this instrument is not available for use now as the manufacturer decided against full-scale production.)

Detection of Neonatal Intracranial Hemorrhage

In 1979 we described a technique for the rapid bedside detection of intracranial hemorrhage in the newborn, utilizing a high-intensity fiberoptic light source and a sensitive cadmium sulfide light meter. This technique takes advantage of the principle that sufficient blood (hemoglobin) will absorb light in the visible wavelength, and by using the anterior fontanelle as a "photo-window," the light meter could detect small quantities of light not absorbed by the cranial contents.

In a separate spectrophotometric study, samples of clear, xanthochromic (nonbloody), and hemorrhagic cerebrospinal fluid were analyzed for absorption spectra. The clear fluid absorbed no appreciable light in the wavelengths detected by the meter (400–650 nm); xanthochromic fluid had a broad absorption band below 520 nm, but no significant absorption between 570 and 750 nm. The grossly bloody fluid had three peaks. The third peak, centered at 577 nm, was sufficient to absorb all of the light in the visible spectrum when the hemoglobin concentration was greater than 0.2 gm/100 ml (derived from Lambert-Beer's law).

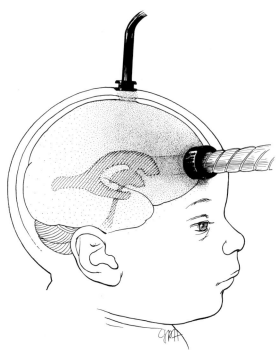

Fig 5–13.—Quantitative cranial transillumination. Schematic drawing showing path of transillumination. Light source is applied to frontal eminence. Light travels through brain and is detected by a sensitive light meter placed over the anterior fontanelle.

The light source used was the Omni-Source fiberoptic light (see chap. 4) with an in-line filter. Its spectral range is from 570 to 750 nm. This technique may be performed without darkening the room, though phototherapy lights and infrared warming lamps should be temporarily discontinued. The light probe is placed on the frontal eminence and directed toward the center of the skull, with the light off. The meter probe is placed directly over the anterior fontanelle and held firmly to avoid light leaks. A baseline meter reading is observed, then the light source is turned on and changes from the baseline are recorded (Fig 5-13). The procedure is then repeated with the light source directed from the opposite frontal eminence. Hemorrhage may be suspected when light transmission fails to occur. These instruments are commercially available now.

In our initial series, 145 infants (birthweights from 850 to 5,300 gm, gestational ages from 27 to 42 weeks) were screened for the presence of hemorrhage. Seventeen failed to transmit light; all were subsequently shown (13 by computed brain tomography, 4 by autopsy) to have intracranial hemorrhage. Nine had intraventricular hemorrhage, 7 had subarachnoid hemorrhage, and 1 had a subarachnoid and unilateral subdural hemorrhage. Seventeen other infants with normal light transmission received definitive central nervous system evaluation (computed brain tomography or autopsy). Sixteen had no evidence of intracranial bleeding; one hemorrhage was present in an infant with massive subcutaneous emphysema of the head and neck. It is probable that the light meter detected subcutaneous light transmission.

This technique cannot distinguish the type of hemorrhage present (e.g., intraventricular vs. subarachnoid), though a unilateral subdural hemorrhage may be suspected. It also appears that an isolated subependymal (germinal matrix) hemorrhage is too small to be diagnosed by this method. Cranial ultrasound is best for this. Quantitative cranial transillumination can be a useful screening tool in infants suspected for intracranial hemorrhage, especially in nurseries where ultrasonography is not available and where accessibility to computed tomographic brain scanners is difficult (though even computed tomography may *not* detect subarachnoid hemorrhage at times).

Other Applications

The reader is referred to the bibliography following this chapter for more complete descriptions of the application of transillumination to other cranial structures. Among the uses reported are transillumination of the optic fundus using a light coagulator (Abrams, 1968); transillumination biomicroscopical examination of the anterior chamber angle and the uvea (Cohen et al., 1976); transocular transcutaneous transillumination in the testing of Bell's phenomenon (Cohen et al., 1977); transillumination of the iris, both infrared (Saari et al., 1978) and visible (Donaldson, 1974); transillumination ophthalmoscopy (Peyman and Sanders, 1975); bright light operative localization (Neubauer, 1968); transillumination to reveal choroidal blood vessels (Freeman and Schepens, 1975); transillumination guidance of subretinal puncture (Dominguez, 1975); use of a fiberoptic conjunctivorhinostomy probe (Sisler, 1976); transillumination of the tympanum (Souri, 1976); fiberoptic transillumination of the sinuses (Binner and Schmidbauer, 1978); and transillumination photography of the eye (Lichter, 1972).

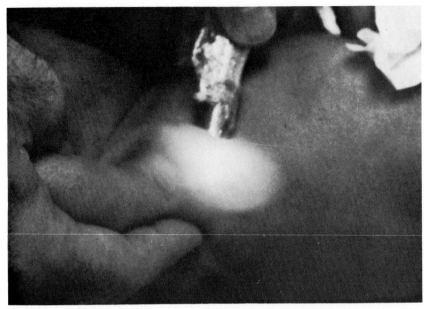

Fig 5–14.—Axillary cystic hygroma. Positive transillumination suggested cystic nature. Ultrasonography confirmed the diagnosis, demonstrating a cystic structure with multiple septae. The axillary location is somewhat less common than the cervicothoracic location usually seen (photograph courtesy of Dr. R.C. Banagale). See also color plate III.

TRANSILLUMINATION OF THE NECK

Cystic hygromas are particularly well evaluated using transillumination. Multiloculated lucent areas are noted within cystic hygromas. After surgery or later in the evolution of a cystic hygroma, there is an increase in the fibrous tissue in the walls, and it is more difficult to see the transillumination. The extent of the cystic hygroma in the supraclavicular region can be evaluated using transillumination (Fig 5-14; color plate III), but it is difficult to evaluate for the extension into the thoracic space, and for this purpose fluoroscopy is required. The cystic hygroma can be injected using transillumination, but only some of the locules fill, and the full extent of the lesion cannot be appreciated after injection of contrast.

Neurofibromas, neuroblastomas, and neurinomas present as neck masses in the cervicothoracic region. We have seen one infant in which palpation by the surgeon indicated that the lesion was a cystic hygroma. However, on transillumination, the mass did not transilluminate, and at surgery a neuroblastoma in the cervicothoracic region was noted. Ultrasonography can be used to delineate the extent of cervicothoracic cystic hygromas; however, it is difficult to obtain contact scans. Real-time scanning is also difficult due to the irregularity of the supraclavicular and neck region, and the difficulty in maintaining contact with the transducer.

With transillumination there is no problem of having to make contact in multiple irregular areas. The transilluminating probe tip can be simply placed over the major palpable mass, most of which will transilluminate if it is a cystic hygroma. We have not been successful in transilluminating branchial cleft cysts, perhaps because of their inflamed and thickened walls. We have also attempted to transilluminate the trachea to aid in proper placement of endotracheal tubes, and this has been unsuccessful. It is possible that a lighted tip could be applied to the end of an endotracheal tube, in which case it would be easy to place the tube in the correct position in the trachea; but, to date, such endotracheal tube lights have not been produced. Posterior encephaloceles and encephalomeningoceles can present at the craniocervical junction. Encephaloceles do not usually transilluminate well. The brain substance does not transilluminate as well as cystic structures. On the other hand, meningoceles in the craniocervical junction do transilluminate well and can be diagnosed using transillumination.

REFERENCES

Abrams, J.D.: Transillumination of the fundus using the light coagulator. *Trans. Ophthalmol. Soc. U.K.* 87:163–169, 1967.

Alexander E., Jr., et al.: Hydranencephaly: Observations on transillumination of the head of infants. *Arch. Neurol. Psychiatr.* 76:578–584, 1956.

Binner W.H., Schmidbauer M.: Fibre-optic transillumination of the sinuses: A comparison of the value of radiography and transillumination in antral disease. *Clin. Otolaryngol.* 3:1–11, 1978.

Buck J.R., et al.: Fiberoptic transillumination: A new tool for the pediatric surgeon. *J. Pediatr. Surg.* 12:451–463, 1977.

Calliauw L.: The value of transillumination of the skull in neurological examination of neonates and infants. *Acta Neurochir.* 10:75–91, 1961.

Cheldelin L.V., et al.: Normal values for transillumination of skull using a new light source. *J. Pediatr.* 87:937–938, 1975.

Cohen S.W., et al.: Biomicroscopical choroidoscopy (uveoscopy) and transillumination gonioscopy. *Arch. Ophthalmol.* 94:1618–1621, 1976.

Cohen S.W., et al.: Testing of Bell's phenomenon by transocular transcutaneous transillumination. *Am. J. Ophthalmol.* 84:735, 1977.

Dodge P.R., Porter P.: Demonstration of intracranial pathology by transillumination. *Arch. Neurol.* 5:30–41, 1961.

Dominquez A.: Puncture of subretinal fluid controlled by transillumination with fiberoptics. *Mod. Probl. Ophthalmol.* 15:134–136, 1975.

Donaldson D.D.: Transillumination of the iris. *Trans Am. Ophthalmol. Soc.* 72:88–106, 1974.

Donn S.M., et al.: Rapid detection of neonatal intracranial hemorrhage by transillumination. *Pediatrics.* 64:843–847, 1979.

Freeman H.M., Schepens C.L.: Innovations in the technique for drainage of subretinal fluid transillumination and choroidal diathermy. *Mod. Probl. Ophthalmol.* 15:119–126, 1975.

Haller J.S.: Skull transillumination, in Coleman M.C. (ed.): *Neonatal Neurology.* Baltimore, University Park Press, 1981.

Hamby W.B., et al.: Hydranencephaly: Clinical diagnosis. *Pediatrics* 6:371–383, 1950.

Hayden P.W., et al.: A pulsed transilluminator for the infant cranium. *Clin. Pediatr.* 14:627–632, 1975.

Horner F.A.: The technique of transillumination of the skull. *Am. J. Dis. Child.* 103:183–185, 1962.

Horner F.A., et al.: Diagnosis of collection of subdural fluid by transillumination. *Am. J. Dis. Child.* 96:594, 1958.

Kuhns L.R., et al.: Transillumination detection of a growing skull fracture. *Am. J. Dis. Child.* 131:889–892, 1977.

Levin J.C.: The value of transillumination in the diagnosis of hydranencephaly. *J. Pediatr.* 50:55–58, 1957.

Lichter P.R.: Transillumination photography of the eye. *Am. J. Ophthalmol.* 73:927–931, 1972.

Mazur R: Transillumination of the skull in the diagnosis of intracranial disease in children up to 3 years. *Dev. Med. Child. Neurol.* 7:634–642, 1965.

Neubauer H.: Intraocular foreign bodies: Bright light operative location. *Int. Ophthalmol. Clin.* 8:205–209, 1968.

Nixon G.W., et al.: Congenital porencephaly. *Pediatrics* 54:43–50, 1974.

Peyman G.A., Sanders D.R.: Transillumination ophthalmoscopy: Instrumentation and technique. *Ophthalmic Surg.* 6:15–16, 1975.

Robinson R.: Transillumination of the head. *Dev. Med. Child. Neurol.* 6:297–299, 1964.

Roessmann U., Parks P.J. Jr.: Hydranencephaly in vertebral-basilar territory. *Acta Neuropathol. (Berl.)* 44:141–143, 1978.

Saari M., et al.: Infra-red transillumination stereophotography of the iris in Fuchs's heterochromic cyclitis. *Brit. J. Ophthalmol.* 62:110–115, 1978.

Shurtleff D.B.: Transillumination. *Perinatal Care* 2:22–25, 1978.

Shurtleff D.B.: Transillumination of skull in infants and children. *Am. J. Dis. Child.* 107:14–24, 1964.

Shurtleff D.B., et al.: Clinical use of transillumination. *Arch. Dis. Child.* 41:183–187, 1966.

Sisler H.A.: Fiberoptic conjunctivorhinostomy probe. *Trans. Am. Acad. Ophthalmol. Otolaryngol.* 81:943–944, 1976.

Sjögren I., Engsner G.: Transillumination of the skull in infants and children. *Acta Paediatr. Scand.* 61:426–428, 1972.

Souri E.: Transillumination of the canine tympanum. *VM. SAC.* 71:302–305, 1976.

Storey B.: Transillumination of the skull in infants and children: A forgotten physical sign? *Med. J. Aust.* 1:491–492, 1968.

Swick H.M., et al.: Transillumination of the skull in premature infants. *Pediatrics* 58:658–664, 1976.

Volpe J.J.: *Neurology of the Newborn*. Philadelphia, W.B. Saunders, 1981.

Vyhmeister N., et al.: Cranial transillumination norms of the premature infant. *J. Pediatr.* 91:980–982, 1977.

Wyman M.L.: Uses of transillumination in the newborn nursery. *Perinatol/Neonatol.* Jan./Feb. 1978.

6

Chest

TRANSILLUMINATION HAS BEEN successfully employed in the diagnosis and treatment of major intrathoracic air leaks. Since alveolar rupture is a relatively common occurrence in the neonatal intensive care unit, and the development of a tension pneumothorax can become a rapidly life-threatening event in the preterm infant, rapid diagnosis and management are obligatory. However, the often subtle clinical presentation of this condition may delay diagnosis until chest radiography is performed. In the setting of a typical neonatal intensive care unit this is often a time-consuming procedure, especially at night, as portable radiographic equipment must be wheeled to the bedside, the patient—often connected to vital life-support systems—must be properly positioned, and the radiograph must be processed. Transillumination has enabled rapid, accurate, noninvasive, bedside diagnosis of pneumothorax, pneumomediastinum, and pneumopericardium. It allows immediate intervention, provides a guide for needle or tube insertion, and allows immediate follow-up and detection of recurrence.

TECHNIQUE

A high-intensity light source is required and the room must be darkened. At night this is easily accomplished, even in units with large windows. Daytime use requires installation of opaque window shades. The light source is filtered and the probe tip is prepared with the rubber sheath, as described earlier. Polyurethane paper (Saran wrap) is placed over the probe to avoid cross-contamination between patients. We cultured ten randomly acquired pieces of Saran wrap and got no growth of pathogenic organisms from any pieces. The infant is placed in the supine position and the light probe is initially positioned supe-

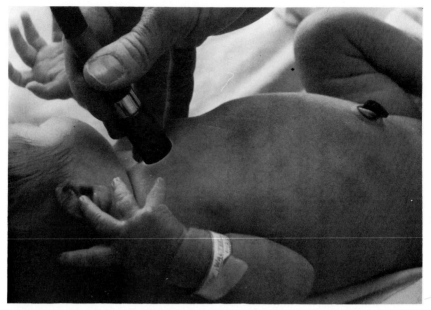

Fig 6–1.—Transillumination of the chest. The light probe is placed in a position superior to the nipple.

rior to one nipple, then activated (Fig 6-1). Normally, a 2- to 3-cm rim of lucency is seen around the probe tip. However, the presence of air in the light path increases the zone of lucency away from this corona which is proportional to the volume of air. Thus, a large unilateral pneumothorax may "light-up" the entire hemithorax (Fig 6-2). A large pneumomediastinum may produce the same result. The probe tip should be moved to various locations on both sides of the chest to complete the procedure. The probe tip should be placed perpendicular to the chest wall and its locations should include the regions superior (above the nipple) (see Fig 6-1), inferior (below the nipple), medial (sternal border) (Fig 6-3), and lateral (axillae and costal margins) (Fig 6-4). If the infant is not symptomatic and the result is positive, radiographic confirmation may be obtained as it is more accurate to quantitate free air volume by radiography. However, in sudden life-threatening pneumothorax or pneumomediastinum, a positive transillumination should be followed by prompt needle aspiration. Transillumination can serve as a guide for thoracentesis, indicating the location of the air, and can demonstrate its response to aspiration. Periodic follow-up will detect recurrences and the possible need for thoracostomy and water-seal drainage.

Pneumomediastinum is suggested rather than pneumothorax if cardiac pulsations are clearly evident in the lucent area (Fig 6-5). We had hoped that transillumination in the lateral decubitus position would help separate pneumomediastinum from pneumothorax. But neither shows an appreciable shift when the patient's position changes, so this is not useful. Large mediastinal gas collections have a tendency to posterior dissection between the diaphragm and parietal pleura and next to the costal margin. This becomes visible with transillumination if the probe is placed next to the costal margin. The probe tip should be placed along the inferior rib cage laterally to detect these. Transillumination is especially useful for needling these collections when they become quite large; by using a light for guidance, one can avoid needling the diaphragm. Large pneumothoraces, on the other hand, generally expand uniformly in an anterior direction; occasionally, after anterior chest tube placement, they can loculate next to the diaphragm.

The reliability of thoracic transillumination to diagnose pneumomediastinum and pneumothorax has been well established. In the initial series, Kuhns et al. (1975) reported the successful diagnosis of 88 of 90 pneumomediastinums or pneumothoraces (two small pneumomediastinums were not appreciated). Wyman and Kuhns (1977) subsequently demonstrated the accuracy of prior transillumination in 126 radiographically proved cases of pneumomediastinum or pneumothorax. In this series, 47 of 50 pneumomediastinums and 73 of 76 pneumothoraces were correctly diagnosed. The three missed pneumomediastinums were considered minimal on chest radiography, with less than 20 cc of air. Among the three missed pneumothoraces were two infants with gross chest wall edema, and a third infant who was born to a diabetic mother and had increased subcutaneous fat. In these cases large pneumothoraces were missed because diffraction of the light in the chest wall may have interfered with intrathoracic transillumination. The increased fat or subcutaneous fluid causes an increased corona of light which may be seen even over the abdomen. When an infant is edematous, the corona of light will be even larger over the dependent portions of the chest and abdomen; this is in contradistinction to pneumothorax or pneumomediastinum, which produces increased light over anterior portions. The accuracy of the method depends on how dark the room can be made, the intensity of the filtered light, and the experience of the observer. If the room cannot be darkened sufficiently in the daytime, the use of a black sheet over the incubator may allow for satisfactory transillumination.

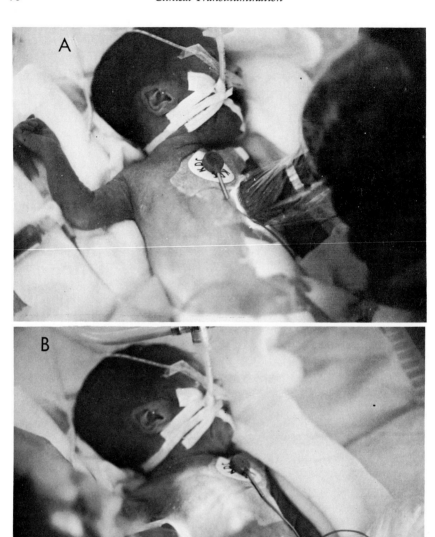

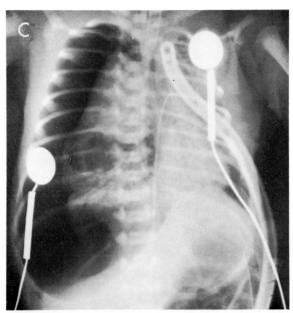

Fig 6–2.—**A,** transillumination of the left chest of a neonate with sudden increased dyspnea. The corona of light around the transilluminator was less wide at this time than it had been during previous transilluminations of the thorax. Tape is seen on the skin just medial to the light, but there was no increased lucency in the area of the tape. **B,** transillumination of the chest in the same neonate. The entire right thoracic cage transilluminated, such that ribs, blood vessels, and the moving right diaphragm can be seen. Note the very lightened paraxiphoid area. **C,** anteroposterior view of the chest obtained after diagnosis by transillumination. A massive right pneumothorax is present. The left chest tube remains from a previous patent ductus arteriosus ligation. (From Kuhns L.R., et al.: Diagnosis of pneumothorax or pneumomediastinum in the neonate by transillumination. *Pediatrics* 56:355–360, 1975. Copyright American Academy of Pediatrics 1975. Used by permission.)

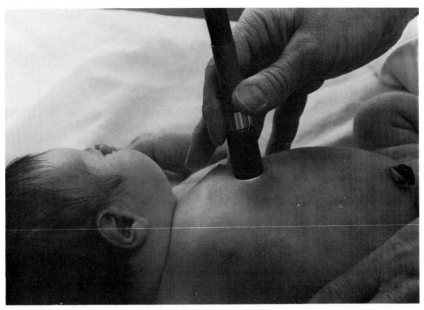

Fig 6–3.—Transillumination of the chest. The light probe is placed in a medial position along the sternal border.

Pneumopericardium is another neonatal emergency that may be detected with transillumination. As for tension pneumothorax, the infant may be too compromised to await radiographic confirmation, and immediate decompression may be indicated. The diagnosis should be suspected from the findings on transillumination. The light probe is placed in the third or fourth intercostal space in the left mid-clavicular line and angled toward the xiphoid process. When the probe is moved over the thorax, the corona of reflected light will become brightest over the area of the pericardial air, and the silhouette of the heartbeat can be seen. (It is not possible in some cases to distinguish pneumomediastinum from pneumopericardium.) Using this as a "target," a 20- or 22-gauge short-bevel 1.5-inch spinal needle without stylet, attached to a 30- or 50-ml syringe may be introduced through a subxiphoid approach, putting gentle negative pressure on the syringe. The pericardial sac is more difficult to puncture than the mediastinum, as it is much more fibrous and requires more force. Entry into the pericardial sac is accompanied by air flow into the syringe and diminution of the

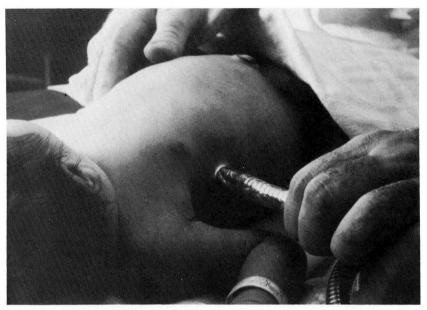

Fig 6–4.—Transillumination of the chest. The light probe is placed in a lateral position along the anterior axillary line.

corona of light at the probe tip; when this occurs the needle is promptly removed to avoid laceration of the coronary vessels. It is advisable to leave a little air in the pericardial sac. Not infrequently needle aspiration provides temporary relief and tube dainage is required. Cabatu and Brown (1979) used this technique to successfully treat three preterm infants with pneumopericardium and encountered no complications of pericardiocentesis (Fig 6-6). We have used it in seven cases without complication.

Transillumination has also been shown to be of benefit in the postoperative management of diaphragmatic hernia. The contralateral hemithorax, which contains the major functional lung tissue, may be serially and frequently monitored for the presence of air leak, thus saving the patient considerable x-ray exposure. The pneumothorax on the operated side can also be followed serially. Large diaphragmatic hernias with bowel loops in the chest will not transilluminate. We have observed this in five cases.

Abnormal accumulations of pleural fluid (hydrothorax or chylo-

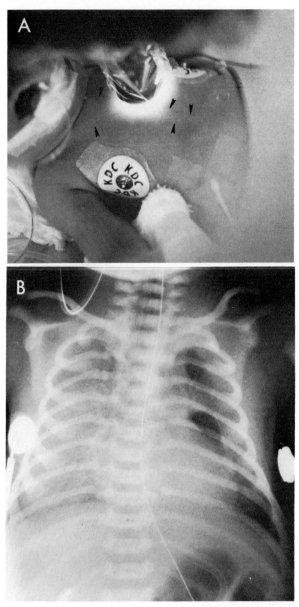

Fig 6–5.—**A,** moderate pneumomediastinum in preterm infant diagnosed by transillumination. Arrowheads indicate linear accumulation of retrosternal air separated from the light probe corona. **B,** anteroposterior radiograph of the same infant taken shortly after transillumination, showing presence of mediastinal air and absence of intrapleural air.

thorax) may be diagnosed by transillumination. We have had several cases in which positive transillumination has led to needle aspiration, but with surprising results, as fluid and not air was removed.

An additional application of thoracic transillumination has been the intraoperative diagnosis of ventricular septal defects. A fiberoptic light source was introduced into one of the ventricles and the ventricular septum was illuminated. The contralateral ventricle was observed for light leaks, indicating defects in the ventricular septum and aiding in their closure (Bernhard et al., 1962; Daneshwar et al., 1979).

Transillumination has also been used in the practice of gynecology as an aid in the diagnosis of breast lesions. Pathologic conditions presenting abnormally on transillumination include benign solid tumor (fibroadenoma), intracystic papilloma, ductal carcinoma, mastitis, cysts, abscesses, galactoceles, hematomas, and pulmonary metastases (Cutler, 1929).

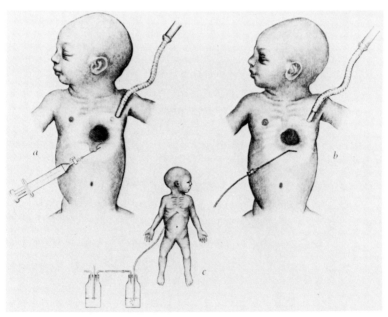

Fig 6–6.—Procedure to illuminate pericardial air: needle aspiration of pneumopericardium *(a)*, catheter in pericardial sac inserted through a Touhy needle *(b)*, and pericardial catheter attached to controlled suction *(c)*. (From Cabatu E.E., Brown E.G.: Thoracic transillumination: Aid in the diagnosis and treatment of pneumopericardium. *Pediatrics* 64:958–960, 1979. Copyright American Academy of Pediatrics 1979. Used by permission.)

REFERENCES

Bernhard W.F., et al.: Transillumination of the ventricular septum: A method for the detection of multiple occult septal defects. *N. Engl. J. Med.* 267:909–912, 1962.

Buck J.R., et al.: Fiberoptic transillumination: A new tool for the pediatric surgeon. *J. Pediatr. Surg.* 12:451–463, 1977.

Cabatu E.E., Brown E.G.: Thoracic transillumination: Aid in the diagnosis and treatment of pneumopericardium. *Pediatrics* 64:958–960, 1979.

Cutler M.: Transillumination as an aid in the diagnosis of breast lesions. *Surg. Gynecol. Obstet.* 48:721–729, 1929.

Daneshwar A., et al.: Transventricular illumination. *Ann. Thorac. Surg.* 28:94–95, 1979.

Kuhns L.R., et al.: Diagnosis of pneumothorax or pneumomediastinum in the neonate by transillumination. *Pediatrics* 56:355–360, 1975.

Wyman M.L.: Uses of transillumination in the newborn nursery. *Perinatol./Neonatol.* Jan./Feb. 1978.

Wyman M.L., Kuhns L.R.: Accuracy of transillumination in the recognition of pneumothorax and pneumomediastinum in the neonate. *Clin. Pediatr.* 16:323–324, 1977.

7

Transillumination of the Abdomen

TRANSILLUMINATION OF THE ABDOMEN can lead to visualization of intra-abdominal structures when the abdominal wall is sufficiently thin. In a child over 2 or 3 years of age, transillumination of the abdomen is usually not successful unless the patient is quite thin and emaciated. On the other hand, transillumination of the abdomen in newborns, especially the premature, can almost always lead to visualization of intra-abdominal viscera (Mofenson and Greensher, 1968; Buck et al., 1977). Severe abdominal wall edema, as in hydropic newborns, prevents visualization of intra-abdominal organs, since the light is diffused by the edema (Fig 7-1). This can be suspected by transillumination because more dependent portions are more susceptible to transillumination (Wyman, 1978). The subcutaneous edema in hydropic infants tends to be most pronounced in the dependent portions of the abdomen, especially the costovertebral angle regions, and can be mistaken for cystic renal structures. This makes visualization of renal structures very difficult in hydropic infants. In adults who are undergoing gastroscopy, colonoscopy, or bronchoscopy, the lighted end of the endoscope can be visualized through the abdominal or chest wall. Since the light has to pass only one way through the abdominal wall to be visualized, light transmission is quite efficient. It is possible that, in the future, transillumination of the abdomen will be feasible in patients of all ages using fiberoptic light sources placed in the colon or stomach.

A fiberoptic light probe is extremely helpful in transillumination of the abdomen. The tip of the fiberoptic probe can be used much as the tip of the palpating finger of the examiner is used in order to place the

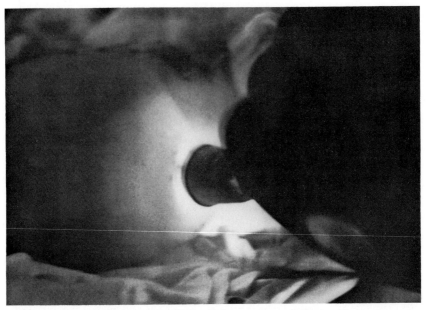

Fig 7–1.—Transillumination of the abdomen in an infant with nonimmune hydrops fetalis. Infant is supine, his head to the left. Chun Gun tip is placed over right lower quadrant. Note diffuse halo of light and failure to discern any of the abdominal viscera.

probe tip near pathologic structures within the abdomen (Fig 7-2). This enhances the success rate of transillumination markedly. The probe tip can be made quite small so that it covers a very small area, which also enhances visualization of viscera.

ABDOMINAL AND PELVIC STRUCTURES

Hollow Viscus Transillumination

In the neonate or young infant who has just been fed, enough air is swallowed for the stomach to be almost always visualized when the probe tip is placed in the left upper quadrant. Patients with hypertrophic pyloric stenosis will have large, gas-distended stomachs at all times, even if they have not eaten recently. Mofenson and Greensher (1968) noted that the entire stomach will transilluminate normally during the first year of life. This distended stomach should not be mistaken for a dilated hydronephrotic kidney or a multicystic kidney, since

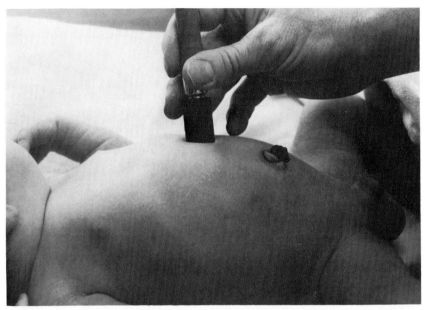

Fig 7–2.—Technique of abdominal transillumination. Tip of fiberoptic light is placed over abdomen and used to gently "probe" the abdominal contents.

renal structures are usually best transilluminated from anterior to posterior with visualization of the abnormal transillumination in the costovertebral region. We have attempted, unsuccessfully, to visualize the abnormal pylorus in hypertrophic pyloric stenosis through the gas-distended stomach using transillumination. Schaff-Blass, Kuhns, and Wyman (1976) used gastric air insufflation as an aid to placement of oral-duodenal tubes. When an orogastric tube is present with the tip in the stomach, insufflation of air produces a large gas-distended stomach which can be easily visualized using transillumination. We found that the distended stomach allows ready passage of a tube around the greater curvature of the stomach into the duodenum since the gastric folds are flattened when the stomach is gas-distended. The tube itself could not be visualized in the gas-distended stomach. When the tip reached the duodenum, insufflation produced visible transillumination of small bowel loops. Nineteen consecutive duodenal intubations were attempted, using two tubes and gastric insufflation; 18 of the attempts were immediately successful. Fifteen attempts in other neonates without gastric insufflation were attempted, and only 1 duodenal intubation was immediately successful.

The small intestine will transilluminate in most neonates and young infants when it is filled with gas. Usually sufficient gas is swallowed to allow visualization of intestinal small bowel loops at almost any time in the neonate. Continuous observation of these loops during transillumination will show peristaltic waves changing the shape of the loops continuously. The duodenum is not visible on transillumination since it is a retroperitoneal structure and is not accessible to the transilluminating probe tip. The colon will also transilluminate when gas-filled. Most neonates and young infants have gas-filled colons at most times. We have not found it possible to differentiate colon from small bowel on the basis of transillumination. These small and large bowel loops can be mistaken for urine-filled, markedly dilated ureters in patients with obstructive uropathy. It can be very difficult at times to know whether one is dealing with dilated ureters or normal bowel loops. Repeated transillumination of the abdomen at different times is helpful, since bowel loops change in configuration and location whereas ureters remain relatively constant in size and shape. However, it is our opinion that other diagnostic imaging techniques should be used to visualize ureters when transillumination suggests ureteral dilatation.

Enteroceles that occur after gynecologic surgery have been successfully transilluminated and diagnosed using transillumination (Altchek, 1965). Rectoceles and rectovaginal fistulas can be detected in this way. Altchek observed that when a light source was placed in the rectum and vaginal inspection was performed using a speculum, the intense transillumination from rectum through posterior vaginal wall occurred normally. Presence of an enterocele masked this bright rectal transillumination. Altchek also used a light source placed in the bladder to visualize the vesicovaginal wall to help assess the extent of fibrosis around vesicovaginal fistulas prior to repair (1962). The extent of fibrosis was visualized directly in this way, which was an important factor in success of repair of the vesicovaginal fistula.

Liver, Gallbladder, and Spleen

The liver can be visualized by placing the fiberoptic probe tip beneath the liver edge just below the right costal margin in the neonate or young infant. Bowel loops beneath the liver edge transilluminate and allow detection of the opaque edge. In the presence of ascites, the liver edge can also be detected. The gallbladder can often be detected in the normal newborn along the anterior inferior edge of the liver

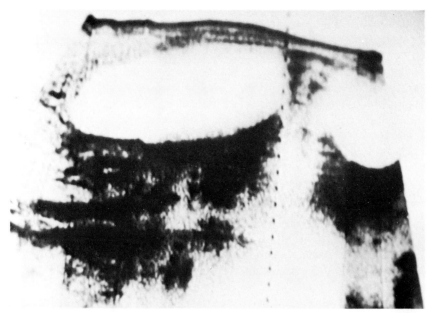

Fig 7–3.—Abdominal ultrasound obtained after abnormal transillumination of the abdomen (see color plate VI). This confirmed the diagnosis of hydrops of the gallbladder.

when intestinal loops are filled with air or ascites is present. However, the gallbladder may be contracted and not visualized along the liver edge. In the patient with marked ascites, transillumination can be helpful in detecting the liver edge even when it is not palpable to help assess and follow liver size. We have not had the opportunity to detect liver cysts using transillumination. In two children with acute hydrops of the gallbladder, we were successful in detecting one very enlarged hydropic gallbladder in a 2-year-old child (color plate V). This diagnosis was subsequently confirmed by ultrasound (Fig 7-3). The gallbladder appeared as a lighted, orange structure despite the green color of the bile within it. The hydrops was not detected in the second, older child due to the thickness of the abdominal wall.

The spleen can occasionally be visualized along the greater curvature of the stomach when the stomach is gas-distended and when the probe tip is placed in the left upper quadrant. In the presence of ascites, the spleen can also be visualized within the ascitic fluid. The medial edge of the spleen is quite lobulated. This can be helpful occasionally in determining whether a neonate or young infant has asplenia. In one neonate with duodenal atresia and a markedly distended stomach, the spleen was visualized anterior and lateral to the stomach. At first we thought this patient had a markedly dilated hydronephrotic kidney, but on subsequent ultrasound examination, this was proved to be a dilated fluid-filled stomach. In this case, the visualization of the spleen along the greater curvature of the abnormally transilluminating mass should have been quite helpful in identifying the structure as stomach rather than hydronephrotic kidney. Renal parenchyma is usually not visualized at all when the kidney is marked hydronephrotic. The spleen tip is multilobulated and has a pancake appearance in contrast to the pear-shaped kidney.

Kidney, Ureter, Bladder, and Scrotum

Transillumination has been used for many years to detect abnormalities of the urinary system (Mofenson and Greensher, 1968; Buck et al., 1977). Urinary cystic and obstructive abnormalities can be evaluated quite well using transillumination in the neonate and young infant (Mofenson and Greensher, 1968). To transilluminate the kidney region, the patient is placed in a decubitus position. The tip of the fiberoptic probe has the opaque cuff removed. The tip of the probe then can be placed deep into the upper quadrant of the side of the abdomen which is highest above the table top (Fig 7-4). The probe tip acts much as a palpating finger during attempted palpation of the kidneys in neonates. The patient's legs can be flexed to relax the abdominal wall. Soft, gentle pressure is applied to the probe until the probe tip is in the region of the kidney. Most bowel loops will be displaced away from the probe tip, but if there is agenesis of the kidney, bowel loops can occupy the renal fossa and simulate a hydronephrotic kidney (Fig 7-5). The examiner then looks at the costovertebral angle from the posterior side of the patient and attempts to determine whether or not an abnormal area of transillumination exists which might suggest a cystic or obstructive lesion of the kidney (color plate VI). Cystic renal structures show with each breath a respiratory excursion which is greater than bowel loop excursion. Occasionally a normal kidney outline itself can be seen when a large amount of bowel gas is present anterior to the kidney. Usually the kidney cannot be visualized when it is within normal limits.

We do not recommend trying to evaluate the kidneys with the patient in the supine position, since bowel loops may simulate renal fluid-filled structures, and the size of renal fluid-filled structures must be quite large to be visualized by transillumination through the anterior

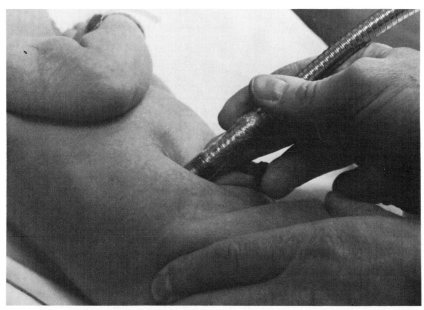

Fig 7–4.—Transillumination technique for the kidney. Patient is placed on the left side. Probe tip is directed into the right hypochondriac area and pressed toward the kidney. The examiner looks at the right costovertebral angle region for abnormal lucency.

abdominal wall. Differentiation of a multicystic kidney (color plate VII) from a hydronephrotic kidney (color plate VI) is not possible, but detection of abnormal fluid collections is quite accurate.

Transillumination can be used to puncture the cystic area, inject contrast, and differentiate hydronephrotic from multicystic kidneys. We transilluminated the kidney region in a series of 30 young infants less than 3 months of age who underwent excretory urography. Seven were found to have obstructed, hydronephrotic kidneys, upper pole duplications with obstruction, or multicystic kidneys. All seven abnormalities were detected by transillumination. Infantile polycystic kidneys (Potter type I) did not produce any abnormal transillumination findings. Within the first year of life, many cystic renal structures (color plate VIII) can still be visualized by transillumination if the patient is cooperative and not excessively obese. Beyond 1 year of age it is difficult to evaluate any part of the urinary tract using transillumination. Visualization of a dilated ureter by transillumination in the anterior and inferior portion of the abdomen when the light is placed anteriorly on

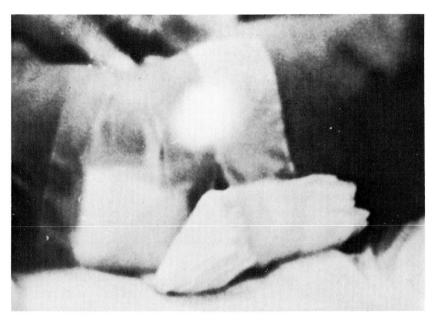

Fig 7–5.—Agenesis of the right kidney with positive transillumination because of the presence of bowel loops in the renal fossa. At surgical exploration for a left ureteropelvic junction obstruction, agenesis of the right kidney was confirmed.

the abdomen is helpful, but bowel loops filled with air or fluid may simulate a dilated ureter.

The bladder can be evaluated by transillumination in essentially all neonates. The probe tip with a rubber sheath on it is placed in the suprapubic region on each side of the rectus muscle and directed toward the midline (Fig 7-6). The bladder appears as a midline translucency. In older children it becomes progressively more difficult to visualize, especially beyond 1 year of age. In a study comparing the height of the bladder as determined by transillumination with the height of the bladder as seen on a simultaneous excretory urogram film in young infants, we found that there was good correlation between transillumination bladder size and excretory urography findings (Kuhns, 1977). This is helpful in evaluating bladder fullness for a suprapubic puncture. If the bladder is empty, obviously the puncture should not be attempted. If the bladder is full, the needle may be directed using transillumination. Often the patient voids as the needle touches the bladder wall, and the transillumination pattern is lost at that point. In

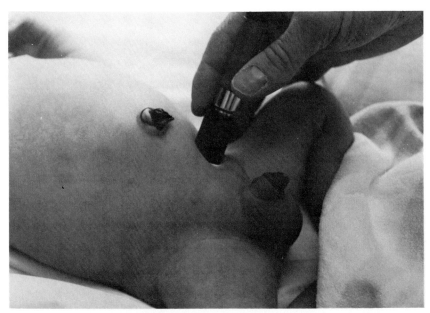

Fig 7–6.—Technique of bladder transillumination. Light probe is placed over suprapubic region on the side of the rectus muscle and directed toward the midline.

neonates and young infants with obstructive uropathy, urethral catheter drainage of the bladder will lead to a decrease in transillumination of the kidneys in the flanks, ureters in the anterior part of the abdomen, and bladder in the suprapubic region. As these structures decrease in visualization under transillumination, it can be determined that the point of obstruction is the bladder or urethra. Catheter drainage can be initiated prior to excretory urography or voiding cystourethrography. Sometimes severely hydronephrotic kidneys do not drain well when the catheter is first placed in the bladder and several days must elapse before the abnormal transilluminating pattern from the hydronephrotic kidney disappears. We have also utilized transillumination of the flank in order to puncture the dilated collecting system of the kidney to perform antegrade pyelography. This is useful in the evaluation of ureteropelvic junction obstructions. We have not been able to transilluminate adrenal cysts successfully.

The scrotum has been examined by transillumination since the time of Bright. It has no subcutaneous fat so that transmission transillumination is possible at all ages. Tumors and hydroceles were classically

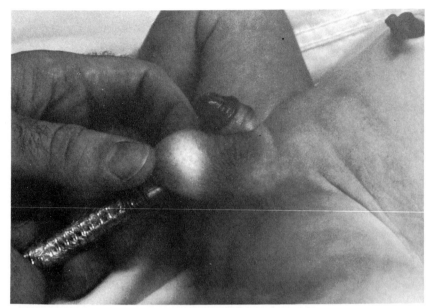

Fig 7–7.—Transillumination demonstration of left hydrocele. Increased lucency results from collection of fluid secondary to a patent processus vaginalis.

diagnosed by transillumination. Today, high resolution ultrasonography has proved more reliable than transillumination in the detection of small testicular tumors. In children, the most common malignancy involving the testes is leukemia, which may recur first in the testicle after a long period of remission. We have been unsuccessful in de tecting testicular changes in leukemia with transillumination. Hydroceles and inguinal hernias are more frequent diagnostic problems in children, and they are readily detected by transillumination. The fluid-filled hydrocele (Fig 7-7) and the fluid- or air-filled intestine in the scrotum both readily transilluminate. We transilluminated a series of 15 children with hydroceles and emptied the hydrocele by digital compression. The ease with which the hydrocele empties depends on the processus vaginalis being patent. Thus, we could predict whether the processus vaginalis was patent or not. At surgery, each of the children whose hydroceles emptied easily under transillumination had patent processus vaginalis communications with the peritoneal space, but we could not predict the size of the opening using compression and transillumination.

Ascites

When the transilluminating probe tip is placed on the anterior abdominal wall, clear ascites within the peritoneal space produces a uniform glow of the anterior abdominal wall (Mofenson and Greensher, 1968; Wyman, 1978). The glow from ascites is less bright than the glow from a pneumoperitoneum. In ascites, the liver edge, gallbladder, and spleen can all be visualized. The falciform ligament can also be seen if the light is placed on the left side of the falciform ligament and the probe tip is pushed deep into the peritoneal space and one looks at the abdomen from the right side. This same sign also is seen in pneumoperitoneum, however. We have utilized transillumination to follow the degree of ascites in neonates. We have been unsuccessful in attempting to evaluate for ascites as a sign of perforation in necrotizing enterocolitis.

Pneumoperitoneum

Pneumoperitoneum, usually due to gastric perforation, perforation from necrotizing enterocolitis, or transdiaphragmatic air leaks, produces a very bright area of abnormal transillumination in the anterior abdomen (Wyman and Kuhns, 1976). Usually the falciform ligament is easily seen as an opaque band running across the area of abnormal glow (color plate IV). One should place the probe tip just to the left of the falciform ligament, push it deep, and look at the abdomen from the right side in order to visualize the falciform ligament (Fig 7-8). Visualization of the falciform ligament is very helpful in determining that the abnormal transillumination is due to pneumoperitoneum rather than bowel loops. The anterior liver edge can sometimes be seen outlined by the pneumoperitoneum, but is not seen as well as in ascites, since the air pushes the liver posteriorly as it accumulates in the peritoneum, whereas ascitic fluid surrounds the liver and spleen but does not displace them posteriorly.

The free air does not enter the flank regions and produce the abnormal glow there that ascites does. However, ascites may coincide with pneumoperitoneum after hollow viscus perforation, and, in that case, there is a glow in the flanks which is more faint than that due to the gas in the anterior abdomen (see Fig 7-1). It is possible to follow neonates with necrotizing enterocolitis for development of a pneumoperitoneum using transillumination; pneumoperitoneum is easily detected. The umbilical vessels can be visualized between the umbilicus and the pubic bone when a large pneumoperitoneum is present (Altchek, 1975).

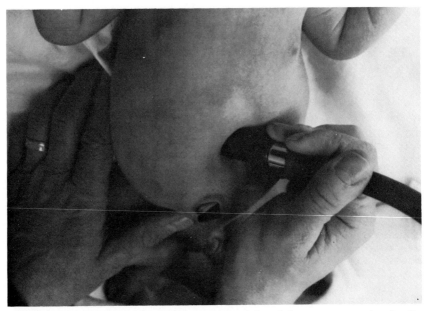

Fig 7–8.—Technique of transillumination of the abdomen to examine for the presence of free air (pneumoperitoneum). Place the probe tip just to the left of the falciform ligament, push it deep, and look at the abdomen from the right side. See color plate IV.

The medial and lateral umbilical ligaments are visualized using transillumination when the pneumoperitoneum extends into the suprapubic region.

TRANSILLUMINATION OF THE SPINE

Transillumination of the spine has proved most useful in our hands in the evaluation of spinal dysraphism. Children with meningocele, meningomyelocele, or a lipomeningocele can be evaluated using transillumination. The probe tip is placed on each side of the soft tissue defect overlying the lower spine. Meningoceles transilluminate very well. Lipomatous elements and teratomatous elements that can occur within the soft tissue mass overlying the spine do not transilluminate as well. Sometimes nerve roots may be seen coursing through the meningomyelocele. In patients with lipomeningoceles, a more translucent portion is seen which represents the meningocele, whereas the fatty elements will also transilluminate but not as brightly as the cystic ele-

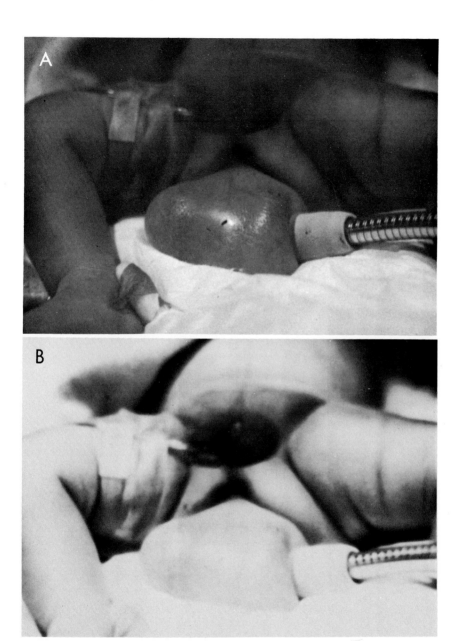

Fig 7–9.—A, newborn infant with sacral mass. Probe tip is placed on the left side of the mass. **B,** after activation of light the cystic areas in the mass glow brightly, solid components appear as darker areas within the mass. At least two histologic components were predicted to be present. The pathologic diagnosis was sacrococcygeal teratoma.

ments. One can thus predict to some degree the contents of these soft tissue masses in spinal dysraphism.

Sacrococcygeal teratomas can also be evaluated using transillumination. The mass can be predicted to be cystic or solid, or a combination of the two (Fig 7-9). The extent of the sacrococcygeal teratoma is important in the preoperative evaluation. When a sacrococcygeal teratoma is largely cystic, the probe tip can be placed on the teratoma, and a glow within the pelvis is noted if the tumor extends into the pelvis.

REFERENCES

Altchek A.: Diagnosis of enterocele by negative intrarectal transillumination. *Obstet. Gynecol.* 26:636–639, 1965.

Altchek A.: Transillumination—a new method of vesicovaginal fistula investigation. *Obstet. Gynecol.* 20:458–461, 1962.

Buck J.R., et al.: Fiberoptic transillumination: A new tool for the pediatric surgeon. *J. Pediatr. Surg.* 12:451–463, 1977.

Kuhns L.R.: Bladder transillumination to facilitate bladder puncture. *J. Pediatr.* 91:850, 1977.

Mofenson H.C., Greensher J.: Transillumination of the abdomen in infants. *Am. J. Dis. Child.* 115:428–431, 1968.

Schaff-Blass E., et al.: Gastric air insufflation as an aid to placement of oroduodenal tubes. *J. Pediatr.* 89:954–955, 1976.

Wyman M.L.: Uses of transillumination in the newborn nursery. *Perinatol./ Neonatol.* Jan./Feb., 1978.

Wyman M.L., Kuhns L.R.: Pneumoperitoneum demonstrated by transillumination. *Am. J. Dis. Child.* 130:1237–1238, 1976.

8

Extremities and Vessels

VASCULAR APPLICATIONS

Transillumination has been a useful adjunct in the location of vascular structures for percutaneous blood sampling or cannulation. This is especially useful in the low birth weight infant where the importance of monitoring arterial blood gases is well established and where arterial and venous access may be difficult because of the infant's size.

The technique for infant venipuncture may also be applied to older children, especially if they are obese, as the light source will transilluminate the subcutaneous fat allowing better visualization of the veins. The veins of the dorsal or volar surface of the wrist (Fig 8-1), hand (Fig 8-2), or foot (Fig 8-3) are particularly well suited for this procedure since the wrist may be dorsiflexed and the light source held directly beneath the hand or foot (Fig 8-4). Medium-bright room lighting is preferred. When the transilluminator is activated, many small superficial veins become visible and can accommodate needles 23 gauge or smaller (Fig 8-5,A, B). Venous spasm may also be visualized by transillumination when the vein is punctured and may prevent inadvertent needle withdrawal. Inject normal saline, watch the vein turn white (Fig 8-5,C). If the needle tip is subcutaneous, a small white spot will be seen. One can still see the vein and enter it. The procedure may also be applied to the dorsum of the hand, and the feet (for use in inferior venacavography). We have found that the use of an assistant is invaluable in immobilizing the extremity and maintaining contact with the light source. Moreover, this enables the operator to use both hands in performing the venipuncture. However, immobilization can be performed utilizing an armboard splint, and the flexible fiberoptic light source can

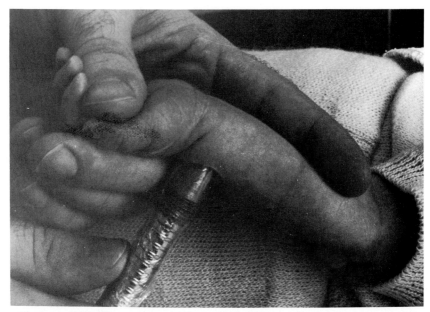

Fig 8–1.—Transillumination of the wrist for venipuncture in a newborn. The hand is slightly extended and the light probe is held against the dorsal wrist surface.

be bent into the proper position if an assistant is unavailable. This procedure is especially useful for dark-skinned people, but works just as well in light-skinned individuals. In older children, place the transilluminator probe on the volar wrist surface and needle the veins on it.

Arterial sampling and cannulation is often a difficult procedure to perform on a sick infant, especially if the pulse is diminished; however, transillumination has allowed visualization of arteries and successful cannulation in even the tiniest and sickest infants. Both the radial and posterior tibial arteries are well suited for this procedure. The technique is essentially the same as that for venipuncture: the wrist or foot is secured and the light source is directed to shine from beneath the extremity (Fig 8-6). In restraining the limbs, care must be taken to avoid a tourniquet effect and diminishing pulsations. Normally the arteries are easily identified by pulsations: they are less well defined than the veins and not as blue. Once located, puncture or cannulation is made under direct visualization. Wall and Kuhns (1977) reported a success rate of 96% (24 of 25) for arterial sampling using this technique,

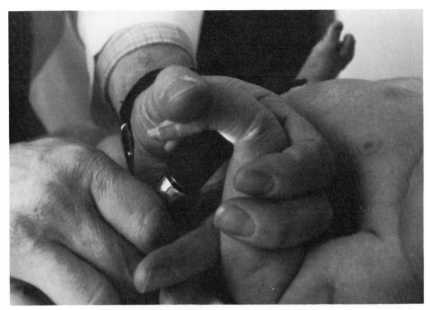

Fig 8–2.—Transillumination of the hand for venipuncture in a newborn. The hand is dorsiflexed over the light source.

applied to the radial (16), ulnar (4), posterior tibial (2), and dorsalis pedis (2) arteries. This was in contrast to a 72% success rate without transillumination. Pearse (1978) reported a 69% (74 of 107) success rate for radial artery catheterization with transillumination and Cole, Todres, and Shannon (1978) reported an 88% (30 of 34) success rate using a similar technique.

Two precautions should always be taken before attempting these procedures. First, care must be taken to avoid thermal injury during these procedures. The light source is likely to be in contact with the patient's skin for a longer period of time than in simple diagnostic transillumination. This requires the filtration of the light (see chap. 3). Turn off the light immediately after entering the vessel. Second, the adequacy of collateral circulation to the hand must be established prior to radial artery cannulation. This may be done by a modification of the Allen test. This involves passively clenching the infant's hand and simultaneous compression of the ulnar and radial arteries. If the entire hand flushes when the ulnar artery is released, collateral circulation is adequate and the radial artery may be cannulated. However, if blanch-

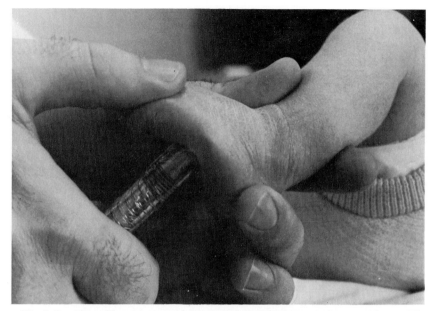

Fig 8–3.—Transillumination of the foot for venipuncture in a newborn. The light source is held against the plantar surface and directed at an oblique angle to transilluminate superficial veins along the lateral aspect of the foot.

ing remains in the distribution of the radial artery after the ulnar artery has been released, insufficient collateral flow exists and the radial artery is unsuitable for cannulation. The size of the arteries may also be assessed by transillumination.

One other vascular application of transillumination has been reported. Percutaneous orbital venography is more easily accomplished when the angular and frontal veins are transilluminated (Cohen et al., 1975). Additionally, delineation of the angular vein aids the ophthalmologist during lacrimal sac surgery.

EXTREMITY LESIONS

In young neonates the probe tip may be placed on either the dorsal or the volar surface of the extremity. Both reflection and transmission transillumination can be evaluated. Extremity lesions which have been most successfully evaluated by us have included cystic or fat-filled lesions. Both types of lesions transilluminate very nicely. Lipomas are

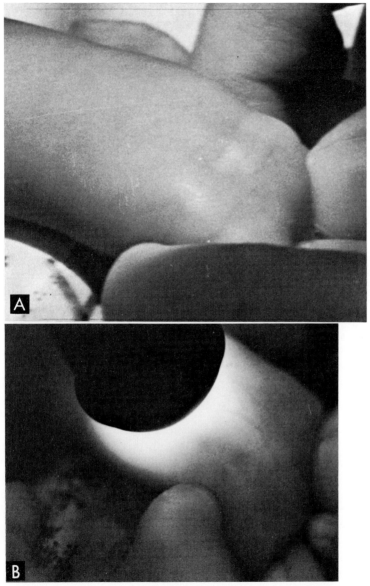

Fig 8–4.—**A,** volar view of dorsiflexed wrist of a 3-week-old infant under room light. **B,** same view of wrist with the transilluminating light applied just above the wrist creases. Note the many small veins. (From Kuhns L.R., et al.: Intense transillumination for infant venipuncture. *Radiology* 116:734–735, 1975. Used by permission.)

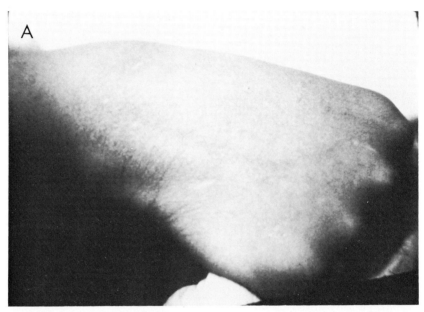

Fig 8–5.—**A,** dorsum of hand of an older child. Note absence of visible veins. **B,** application of intense light source to dorsum of hand of the same child. Note the two large veins at the right edge of the corona *(arrowheads).* **C,** under transillumination guidance venipuncture is made with 21-gauge scalp vein needle. Note the "white" appearance of the vein following injection of normal saline.

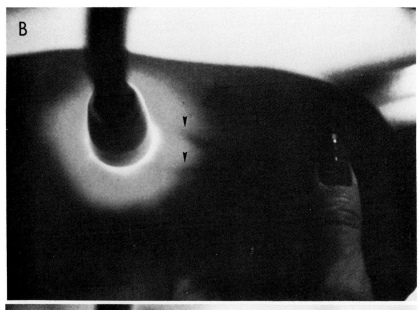

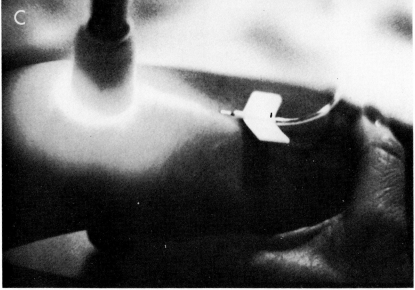

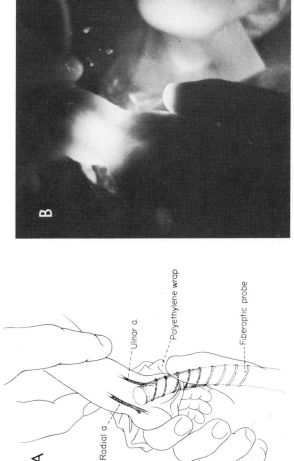

Fig 8-6.—**A,** drawing of positioning of the hand and wrist for radial or ulnar artery puncture. The wrist is dorsiflexed and immobilized over the probe tip. The volar aspect of the wrist is thus exposed. (From Wall P.M., Kuhns L.R.: Percutaneous arterial sampling using transillumination. *Pediatrics* 59 (suppl.): 1032–1035, 1977. Copyright American Academy of Pediatrics 1977. Used by permission.) **B,** transillumination of the wrist for arterial puncture. The radial artery and ulnar artery are seen as linear structures with poorly defined edges due to their pulsations during photography. (From Wall P.M., Kuhns L.R.: Percutaneous arterial sampling using transillumination. *Pediatrics* 59 (suppl.):1032–1035, 1977. Copyright American Academy of Pediatrics 1977. Used by permission.) *(Continued)*

Ulnar a.

Polyethylene wrap

Radial a.

Fiberoptic probe

Fig 8–6 (cont.).—C, drawing of positioning of the ankle for posterior tibial artery puncture. The probe is placed under the lateral malleolus and the ankle is slightly dorsiflexed and everted to immobilize it over the probe tip. (From Wall P.M., Kuhns L.R.: Percutaneous arterial sampling using transillumination. *Pediatrics* 59 (suppl.):1032–1035, 1977. Copyright American Academy of Pediatrics 1977. Used by permission.) **D,** transillumination of the ankle for arterial puncture. The saphenous vein and its tributaries anterior to the medial malleolus are more clearly seen than the posterior tibial artery, due to the darker colored blood in the veins and the lack of venous pulsations. Heel puncture sites are incidentally noted. (From Wall P.M., Kuhns L.R.: Percutaneous arterial sampling using transillumination. *Pediatrics* 59 (suppl.):1032–1035, 1977. Copyright American Academy of Pediatrics 1977. Used by permission.)

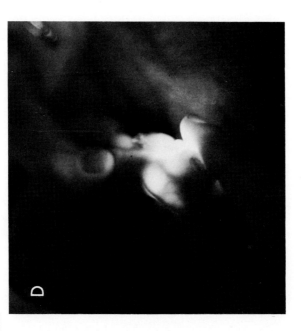

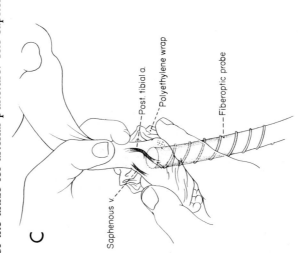

99

easily evaluated by transillumination, as are cystic lesions of the extremities such as cystic hygromas. We have not been successful at transilluminating cystic-filled or fluid-filled joints due to the very dense capsules of the joints. When a lesion of the extremity is hypervascular, a great many veins can be seen around the lesion. This suggests that it is hypervascular and possibly malignant. In one older child, many abnormally dilated veins were noted in the subcutaneous fat of the popliteal region; this child had an arteriovenous malformation of that area. Dermoids of the fingers have been successfully transilluminated.

Digital Mucinous Pseudocysts

This is a lesion which generally occurs on the finger, near the nail, and may be associated with a linear atrophic defect of the nail. L. Goldman et al. (1974) and J.A. Goldman et al. (1977) have described diagnosis of this condition using fiberoptic transillumination. The light probe is directed toward the dorsum of the distal interphalangeal joint. The pseudocyst, because it is mucin-containing, transilluminates.

REFERENCES

Buck J.R., et al.: Fiberoptic transillumination: A new tool for the pediatric surgeon. *J. Pediatr. Surg.* 12:451–463, 1977.

Cohen S.W., et al.: Transillumination of the angular and frontal veins. *Am. J. Ophthalmol.* 80:765–766, 1975.

Cole F.S., et al.: Technique for percutaneous cannulation of the radial artery in the newborn infant. *J. Pediatr.* 92:105–107, 1978.

Feldman B.H.: Arterial cannulation in the newborn infant. *J. Pediatr.* 93:161–162, 1978.

Goldman J.A., et al.: Digital mucinous pseudocysts. *Arthritis Rheum.* 20:997–1002, 1977.

Goldman L., et al.: Transillumination for diagnosis of mucinous pseudocyst of the finger. *Arch. Dermatol.* 109:576, 1974.

Kuhns L.R., et al.: Intense transillumination for infant venipuncture. *Radiology* 116:734–735, 1975.

Pearse R.G.: Percutaneous catheterisation of the radial artery in newborn babies using transillumination. *Arch. Dis. Child.* 53:549–554, 1978.

Stein R.T., et al.: Arterial cannulation in the newborn infant. *J. Pediatr.* 93:162, 1978.

Wall P.M., Kuhns L.R.: Percutaneous arterial sampling using transillumination. *Pediatrics* 59(suppl.):1032–1035, 1977.

Wyman M.L.: Uses of transillumination in the newborn nursery. *Perinatol./Neonatol.* Jan./Feb., 1978.

COLOR PLATES

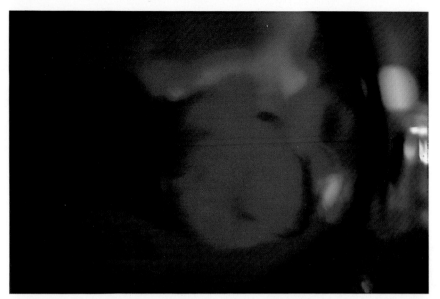

Color Plate I.—Hydrocephalus. Transillumination of the head of a preterm infant with posthemorrhagic hydrocephalus showing generalized increased lucency over the entire skull. Several areas of hemorrhage from previous venipuncture sites can be seen. (From Buck J.R., et al.: Fiberoptic transillumination: A new tool for the pediatric surgeon. *J. Pediatr. Surg.* 12:451–463, 1977. Used by permission.)

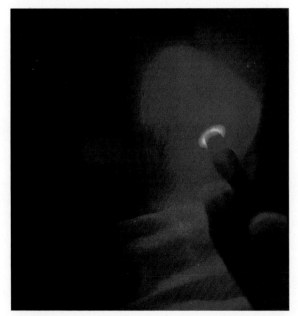

Color Plate II.—Posterior fossa arachnoidal cyst. Transillumination of the posterior skull showing a lobulated pattern of lucency. At the peak of this lobulation is the tentorium cerebelli.

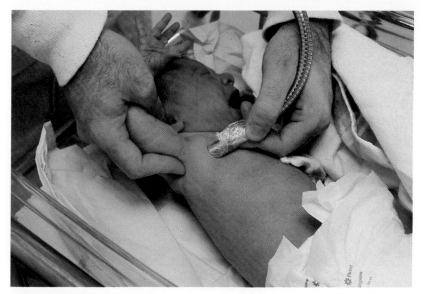

Color Plate III.—Cystic hygroma of the axilla. A large fluctuant axillary mass with a positive transillumination. Diagnosis of cystic hygroma confirmed by ultrasonography (photograph courtesy of Dr. R.C. Banagale).

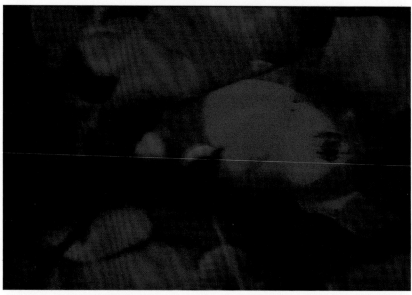

Color Plate IV.—Pneumoperitoneum. Light probe placed over hypogastrium; the entire abdomen glows. The falciform ligament seen anteriorly in the region of the liver. Patient is supine; head is at left.

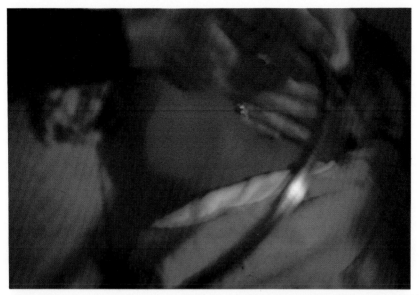

Color Plate V.—Hydrops of the gallbladder. Light probe is placed in a subxiphoid position. The enlarged gallbladder positively transilluminates in the right upper quadrant.

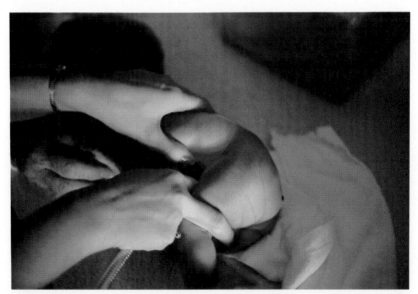

Color Plate VI.—Hydronephrotic left kidney. Grossly positive transillumination is noted over the left flank. Kidney is hydronephrotic secondary to an obstruction at the ureteropelvic junction.

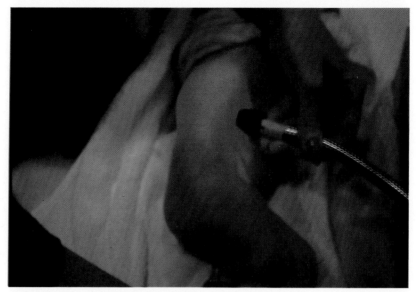

Color Plate VII.—Multicystic right kidney. The kidney failed to visualize on an excretory urogram. The entire right flank glows on transillumination.

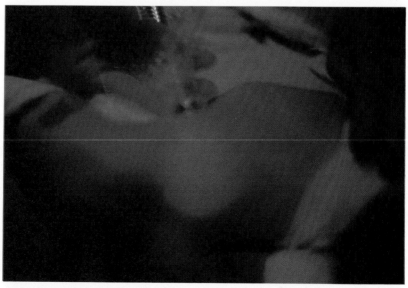

Color Plate VIII.—Simple left renal cyst. Positive transillumination is noted as the infant is viewed from the back.

Part III

APPENDICES

A

Some Physical Aspects of Light

LIGHT, AS WE ordinarily understand it, refers to the portion of the electromagnetic spectrum that we can see. The electromagnetic spectrum includes gamma rays (high energy radiation given off by radioisotopes), x-rays (used by physicians and dentists for diagnostic work), ultraviolet rays (which cause suntan and sunburn), visible light, infrared rays (used for heating food), microwaves (used in microwave ovens), and radio and television waves. Visible light encompasses wavelengths from 400 nm to 700 nm (nm = nanometer = 10^{-9} meter). It is a form of energy and possesses properties that can be explained either by its particulate or by its wave nature.

PROPERTIES OF LIGHT

VELOCITY OF LIGHT.—The velocity of light (C) in a vacuum is 299,792 km/second or 186,282 miles per second. The velocity is the same for all wavelengths over the whole range of the electromagnetic spectrum from gamma rays to radiowaves.

WAVE NATURE OF LIGHT.—Light travels in the form of a wave with crests and troughs. This is supported by the fact that light displays interference and diffraction phenomena which are properties of waves and it also mathematically follows quantum wave mechanics. Light waves may be characterized by either frequency or wavelength. The frequency, v, is the reciprocal of the wavelength, λ, multiplied by the magnitude of the velocity of light, C:

$$v = \frac{C}{\lambda}$$

PARTICULATE NATURE OF LIGHT.—Light consists of tiny particles called photons, which are identified by the amount of their energy (E). The energy of a photon is identified by the equation $E = h\nu$ where h is Planck's constant and ν is the frequency.

PHOTOELECTRIC EFFECT.—When light of suitable frequency falls on a cold alkali metal surface, such as a cathode in diode electronic tube, a current is observed. This current is proportional to the intensity of the illumination. Einstein explained this effect by the particulate nature of light.

INTERFERENCE.—When two or more waves are present, the net effect is calculated by combining the effects of all the waves, the effect of each being calculated as if the other waves were not present.

DIFFRACTION.—If the shadow of an object cast on a screen by a small source of light is examined, it is found that the boundary of the shadow is not sharp. This phenomenon results from light not being propagated strictly in straight lines, but in waves.

MEASUREMENT OF LIGHT

DETECTION OF LIGHT.—Light can be detected visually by the naked eye, electronically by photosensitive vacuum tubes and semiconductors, or photographically by light-sensitive photographic papers.

INTENSITY OF LIGHT.—The unit of intensity measurement is the *lumen*. An obsolete unit of illumination is the foot-candle (ft-c), which is equal to one lumen per square foot.

ENERGY OF LIGHT.—This refers to the wavelength of light (or energy of each photon) that can be measured by a spectrophotometer. The unit of energy can be expressed in wavelength (cm), energy units (electron volts), or frequency (cycles per second, ν).

B

Bibliography

Abrams J.D.: Transillumination of the fundus using the light coagulator. *Trans. Ophthalmol. Soc. U.K.* 87:163–169, 1967.

Alexander E. Jr., et al.: Hydranencephaly: Observations on transillumination of the head of infants. *Arch. Neurol. Psychiatr.* 76:578–584, 1956.

Altchek A.: Diagnosis of enterocele by negative intrarectal transillumination. *Obstet. Gynecol.* 26:636–639, 1965.

Altchek A.: Transillumination—a new method of vesicovaginal fistula investigation. *Obstet. Gynecol.* 20:458–461, 1962.

Bellotti G.A., et al.: Fiberoptic transillumination for intravenous cannulation under general anesthesia. *Anesth. Analg.* 60:348–351, 1981.

Bernhard, W.F., et al.: Transillumination of the ventricular septum. *N. Engl. J. Med.* 267:909–912, 1962.

Binner W.H., Schmidbauer M.: Fibre-optic transillumination of the sinuses: A comparison of the value of radiography and transillumination in antral disease. *Clin. Otolaryngol.* 3:1–11, 1978.

Bokay J.: Die strasburgersche Transparenzuntersuchung bei chronischem Hydrocephalus Internus. *Jahrb. Kinderheilkd.* 78:426–441, 1913.

Bokay J.: Beitrage zur Pathologie und Therapie des chronischen Hydrocephalus Internus. *Jahrb. Kinderheilkd.* 81:17–24, 1915.

Bokay J.: Neue Beitrage zum Wert der Transparenzuntersuchung nach Strasburger bei chronischem Hydrocephalus Internus. *Monatsschr. Kinderheilkd.* 24:43, 1923.

Bokay J.: Über den Wert der Transparenzuntersuchungen bei Hydrocephalus Internus Congenitus. *Acta Paediatr.* 13:48, 1932.

Bomba J.L.: Fiberoptic lighting systems: Their role in dentistry. *Dent. Clin. North Am.* 15:197–218, 1971.

Bright R.: Diseases of the brain and nervous system, in *Reports of Medical Cases Selected With a View of Illustrating the Symptoms and Cure of Diseases by a Reference to Morbid Anatomy.* London, Longman, Rees, Orme, Brown, Green, and Highley, 1831, vol. 2, case ccv.

Brown E.B.: *Modern Optics.* Huntington, New York, R.E. Kreiger, 1974.

Bruck J.: *Das Urethroscop und das Stomatoscop zur Durchleuchtung der Blase und der Zähne und ihrer Nachbartheile durch galvanisches Glühlicht.* Breslau, Maruschke & Berendt, 1867.

Buck J.R., et al.: Fiberoptic transillumination: A new tool for the pediatric surgeon. *J. Pediatr. Surg.* 12:451–463, 1977.

Cabatu E.E., Brown E.G.: Thoracic transillumination: Aid in the diagnosis and treatment of pneumopericardium. *Pediatrics* 64:958–960, 1979.

Calliauw L.: The value of transillumination of the skull in neurological examination of neonates and infants. *Acta Neurochir.* 10:75–91, 1961.

Cambern A.M., et al.: Photography of transilluminated intracranial lesions in infants. *Med. Radiogr. Photogr.* 37:8–11, 1961.

Cameron W.J.: *Diagnosis by Transillumination,* ed 3. Chicago, Cameron's Publishing Co., 1922.

Cheldelin L.V., et al.: Normal values for transillumination of skull using a new light source. *J. Pediatr.* 87:937–938, 1975.

Church S., Adamkin D.H.: Transillumination in neonatal intensive care: A possible iatrogenic complication. *South. Med. J.* 74:76–77, 1981.

Cohen S.W., et al.: Biomicroscopical choroidoscopy (uveoscopy) and transillumination gonioscopy. *Arch. Ophthalmol.* 94:1618–1621, 1976.

Cohen S.W., et al.: Testing of Bell's phenomenon by transocular transcutaneous transillumination. *Am. J. Ophthalmol.* 84:735, 1977.

Cohen S.W., et al.: Transillumination of the angular and frontal veins. *Am. J. Ophthalmol.* 80:765–766, 1975.

Cole F.S., et al.: Technique for percutaneous cannulation of the radial artery in the newborn infant. *J. Pediatr.* 92:105–107, 1978.

Curling T.B.: Hydrocele, in Goddard P.B. (ed.): *A Practical Treatise on the Diseases of the Testis, and of the Spermatic Cord and Scrotum.* Philadelphia, Carey and Hart, 1843, chap. 4.

Cutler M.: Transillumination as an aid in the diagnosis of breast lesions. *Surg. Gynecol. Obstet.* 48:721–729, 1929.

Cutler M.: Transillumination of the breast. *Ann. Surg.* 93:223–234, 1931.

Daneshwar A., et al.: Transventricular illumination. *Ann. Thorac. Surg.* 28:94–95, 1979.

DeGuillebon H., Schepens C.L.: A transilluminator scleral marker. *Arch. Ophthalmol.* 86:298–300, 1971.

Dodge P.R., Porter P.: Demonstration of intracranial pathology by transillumination. *Arch. Neurol.* 5:30–41, 1961.

Dominguez A.: Puncture of subretinal fluid controlled by transillumination with fiberoptics. *Mod. Probl. Ophthalmol.* 15:134–136, 1975.

Donaldson D.D.: Transillumination of the iris. *Trans. Am. Ophthalmol. Soc.* 72:88–106, 1974.

Donn S.M., et al.: Rapid detection of neonatal intracranial hemorrhage by transillumination. *Pediatrics* 64:843–847, 1979.

Donn S.M., et al.: Transillumination—a technical note. *Pediatrics* 66:813–814, 1980.

Feldman B.H.: Arterial cannulation in the newborn infant. *J. Pediatr.* 93:161–162, 1978.

Ford R.J.: Infrared photography of transilluminated infant skulls. *J. Biol. Photogr. Assoc.* 42:94–102, 1974.

Freeman H.M., Schepens C.L.: Innovations in the technique for drainage of subretinal fluid by transillumination and choroidal diathermy. *Mod. Probl. Ophthalmol.* 15:119–126, 1975.

Friedman J., Marcus M.I.: Transillumination of the oral cavity with the use of fiber optics. *J. Am. Dent. Assoc.* 80:801–809, 1970.

Gerbitz S.: Transillumination helps nurses locate veins. *Nursing* 4:12, 1974.

Goldman J.A., et al.: Digital mucinous pseudocysts. *Arthritis Rheum.* 20:997–1002, 1977.

Goldman L.: Transillumination as a diagnostic aid. *Arch. Dermatol.* 112:262, 1976.

Goldman L., et al.: Transillumination for diagnosis of mucinous pseudocyst of the finger. *Arch. Dermatol.* 109:576, 1974.

Haller J.S.: Skull transillumination, in Coleman, M.C. (ed.): *Neonatal Neurology.* Baltimore, University Park Press, 1981.

Hamby W.B., et al.: Hydranencephaly: Clinical diagnosis. *Pediatrics* 6:371–383, 1950.

Hayden P.W., et al.: A pulsed transilluminator for the infant cranium. *Clin. Pediatr.* 14:627–632, 1975.

Hooks V.H., et al.: Focal vascular dysplasia in the cecum demonstrated by intra-operative endoscopic transillumination. *Gastrointest. Endosc.* 25:69–71, 1979.

Horner F.A.: The technique of transillumination of the skull. *Am. J. Dis. Child.* 103:183–184, 1962.

Horner F.A., et al.: Diagnosis of collection of subdural fluid by transillumination. *Am. J. Dis. Child.* 96:594–595, 1958.

Johnson C.C., et al.: Infant cranial transillumination. *Med. Instrum.* 7:62, 1973.

Jonas A.D.: Skull transillumination. *Br. Med. J.* 2(920):671–672, 1974.

Kerker M.: *The Scattering of Light and Other Electromagnetic Radiation.* New York, Academic Press, 1969.

King D.R., King A.C.: Signficance of external light source in diagnosis by fiber optics. *J. Oral. Med.* 30:15, 1975.

Kravitz H., et al.: A technique for improved visualization of the umbilical vessels. *IMJ.* 130:23–25, 1966.

Kuhns L.R.: Bladder transillumination to facilitate bladder puncture. *J. Pediatr.* 91:850, 1977.

Kuhns L.R., et al.: A caution about using photoillumination devices. *Pediatrics* 57:975–976, 1976.

Kuhns L.R., et al.: Diagnosis of pneumothorax and pneumomediastinum in the neonate by transillumination. *Pediatrics* 56:355–360, 1975.

Kuhns L.R., et al.: Intense transillumination for infant venipuncture. *Radiology* 116:734–735, 1975.

Kuhns L.R., et al.: Transillumination detection of a growing skull fracture. *Am. J. Dis. Child.* 131:889–892, 1977.

Lehman R.A.W., et al.: Cystic intracranial teratoma in an infant. *J. Neurosurg.* 33:334–338, 1970.

Leis H.P.: Clinical diagnosis of breast cancer. *J. Reprod. Med.* 14:231–240, 1975.

Levin J.C.: The value of transillumination in the diagnosis of hydranencephaly. *J. Pediatr.* 50:55–58, 1957.

Lichter P.R.: Transillumination photography of the eye. *Am. J. Ophthalmol.* 73:927–931, 1972.

Lim E.C. (ed.): *Excited States.* New York, Academic Press, 1974, vol. 1.

McArtor R.D., Saunders B.S.: Iatrogenic second degree burn caused by a trans-illuminator. *Pediatrics* 63:422–424, 1979.

Martin A.J., et al.: Production of a permanent radiographic record of transillu-mination of the neonate. *Radiology* 122:540–541, 1977.

Mazur R.: Transillumination of the skull in the diagnosis of intracranial disease in children up to 3 years. *Dev. Med. Child. Neurol.* 7:634–642, 1965.

Mofenson H.C., Greensher J.: Transillumination of the abdomen in infants. *Am. J. Dis. Child.* 115:428–431, 1968.

Moore J.G.: Transilluminator using fibre ray lighting. *Br. J. Ophthalmol.* 53:711–713, 1969.

Neubauer H.: Intraocular foreign bodies. Bright light operative localization. *Int. Opthalmol. Clin.* 8:205–209, 1968.

Nixon G.W., et al.: Congenital porencephaly. *Pediatrics* 54:43–50, 1974.

Ochsner A.: Diseases of the breast. *Postgrad. Med.* 57:77–84, 1975.

Paul S.D., Singh K.M.: Differential macular illumination tests. *Ophthalmologica* 160:409–420, 1970.

Pearse R.G.: Percutaneous catheterisation of the radial artery in newborn ba-bies using transillumination. *Arch Dis. Child.* 53:549–554, 1978.

Peyman G.A., Sanders D.R.: Transillumination ophthalmoscopy: Instrumen-tation and technique. *Ophthal. Surg.* 6:15–16, 1975.

Piasecki C.: In vivo transillumination of the submucous plexus of vessels in the dog's stomach. *J. Anat.* 105:210, 1969.

Purdell-Lewis D.J., et al.: A comparison of radiographic and fibre-optic diag-nosis of approximal caries lesions. *J. Dent.* 2:143–148, 1974.

Rabe E.F.: Skull transillumination in infants. *GP* 36:78–88, 1967.

Robinson R.: Transillumination of the head. *Dev. Med. Child. Neurol.* 6:297–299, 1964.

Roessmann U., Parks P.J. Jr.: Hydranencephaly in vertebral-basilar territory. *Acta. Neurophathol. (Berl.)* 44:141–143, 1978.

Rozovski J., et al.: Cranial transillumination in early and severe malnutrition. *Br. J. Nutr.* 25:107–111, 1971.

Saari M., et al.: Infra-red transillumination stereophotography of the iris in Fuchs's heterochromic cyclitis. *Br. J. Ophthalmol.* 62:110–115, 1978.

Scanlon J.W.: A modification of the chest transilluminator. *Pediatrics* 60:766, 1977.

Schaff-Blass E., et al.: Gastric air insufflation as an aid to placement of oro-duodenal tubes. *J. Pediatr.* 89:954–955, 1976.

Sewell I.A.: Recent advances in transillumination techniques. *Bibl. Anat.* 10:549–556, 1969.

Shurtleff D.B.: Transillumination. *Perinatal Care* 2:22–25, 1978.

Shurtleff D.B.: Transillumination of skull in infants and children. *Am. J. Dis. Child.* 107:14–24, 1964.

Shurtleff D.B., et al.: Clinical uses of transillumination. *Arch. Dis. Child.* 41:183–187, 1966.

Shurtleff D.B. et al.: Congenital brain cysts in infancy: Diagnosis, treatment, and follow-up. *Teratology* 7:183–190, 1973.

Simpson J.: A lecture on the Siamese and other viable united twins. *Br. Med. J.* 1:139, 1869.

Sisler H.A.: Fiberoptic conjunctivorhinostomy probe. *Trans. Am. Acad. Ophthalmol. Otolaryngol.* 81:943–944, 1976.

Sjögren I., Engsner G.: Transillumination of skull in infants and children: Recording with a new point scale. *Acta. Paediatr. Scand.* 61:426–428, 1972.

Souri E.: Transillumination of the canine tympanum. *VM. SAC.* 71:302–305, 1976.

Starr M.C., Netto D.J.: A light pipe for the transillumination of hollow organs during in vivo microscopy. *Microvasc. Res.* 6:360–361, 1973.

Storey B.: Transillumination of the skull in infants and children: A forgotten physical sign? *Med. J. Aust.* 1:491–492, 1968.

Strasburger J.: Transparenz des Kopies bei Hydrocephalus. *Dtsch. Med. Wochenschr.* 36:294, 1910.

Swick H.M., et al.: Transillumination of the skull in premature infants. *Pediatrics* 58:658–664, 1976.

Taylor L., et al.: An apparatus for photography of transillumination of the head. *J. Neurosurg.* 13:219–220, 1956.

Taylor R.C. et al.: Illumination of the oral cavity. *J. Am. Dent. Assoc.* 74:1207–1209, 1967.

Tiedt, J.N.: A simple method for transilluminating the maxillary sinuses. *J. Biol. Photogr. Assoc.* 37:117–118, 1969.

Uy J.O., et al.: Light filtration during transillumination of the neonate: A method to reduce heat buildup in the skin. *Pediatrics* 60:308–312, 1977.

Viggiani E.: An apparatus to facilitate light transmission measurements through living tissues. *Bull. Soc. Ital. Biol. Sper.* 54:559–564, 1978.

Volpe J.J.: *Neurology of the Newborn.* Philadelphia, W.B. Saunders, 1981.

Vyhmeister N., et al.: Cranial transillumination norms of the premature infant. *J. Pediatr.* 91:980–982, 1977.

Wall P.M., Kuhns L.R.: Percutaneous arterial sampling using transillumination. *Pediatrics* 59(suppl.):1032–1035, 1977.

Wedge J.J., et al.: Abdominal masses in the newborn: 63 cases. *J. Urol.* 106:770–775, 1971.

Wolter J.R.: Transillumination of enucleated eyes with an egg candler. *Arch. Ophthalmol.* 88:662–663, 1972.

Wright G.Z., et al.: An evaluation of transillumination for caries detection in primary molars. *J. Dent. Child.* 39:199–202, 1972.

Wyman M.L.: Uses of transillumination in the newborn nursery. *Perinatol./Neonatol.* Jan./Feb. 1978.

Wyman M.L., Kuhns L.R.: Accuracy of transillumination in the recognition of pneumothorax and pneumomediastinum in the neonate. *Clin. Pediatr.* 16:323–324, 1977.

Wyman M.L., Kuhns L.R.: Pneumoperitoneum demonstrated by transillumination. *Am. J. Dis. Child.* 130:1237–1238, 1976.

Zervoudakis I.A., Birnbaum S.J.: Transillumination in operative gynecology. *Am. J. Obstet. Gynecol.* 127:209–211, 1977.

Index